JIMMY LOCKETT

You Can Still Move with Ease and Strength at 50, 60, 70 (and Beyond)

Proven Practices to stay Mobile, Strong, Energized, and Independent at Every Age

Copyright © 2025 by Jimmy Lockett

All rights reserved. No part of this publication may be reproduced, stored or transmitted in any form or by any means, electronic, mechanical, photocopying, recording, scanning, or otherwise without written permission from the publisher. It is illegal to copy this book, post it to a website, or distribute it by any other means without permission.

First edition

This book was professionally typeset on Reedsy. Find out more at reedsy.com

Contents

Chapter 1	1
A New Model of Fitness for Aging Well	1
Fit for What?	1
The Longevity Triad	3
Training to Stay Capable	4
The Mind-Body Loop	6
Science Snapshot: Key Takeaways from Chapter 1	7
Chapter 2	10
The Fundamentals of a Fit Life	10
Move Every Day (Baseline Movement Habits)	10
Build and Keep Muscle (Strength & Resistance)	12
Breathe, Push, Recover (Cardio and Conditioning)	13
Balance, Mobility, and Joint Care	15
Recovery as Training	16
Chapter 3	20
The Psychology of Lifelong Fitness	20
The Identity Shift	20
Motivation, Meaning, and Momentum	21
Habit Stacking and Environmental Design	23
Chapter 4	25
The ACF Model – High-Functioning Movement After 50	25
What Is ACF?	25

The 7 ACF Principles Applied to Physical Vitality	27
The ACF Pyramid Applied to Movement	32
Life as Training: A Story-Based Overview	36

Chapter 5 — 39

Testing, Tracking, and Personal Metrics — 39

Where Are You Now? The Importance of Baseline Testing — 39

Useful Metrics (and How to Track Them) — 42

Advanced Assessment Tools — 46

Chapter 6 — 52

Tier 1: Foundation – Daily Movement — 52

Movement is Non-Negotiable — 52

Core Habits for Daily Vitality — 55

Practice Plan: Weeks 1–4 — 59

What You'll Notice — 62

Chapter 7 — 65

Tier 2: Intentional Exercise – Strength and Resilience — 65

The Sweet Spot of Training Intensity — 65

Your Weekly Framework — 68

Practice Plan: Weeks 5–8 — 72

Wins to Look For — 76

Chapter 8 — 79

Tier 3: Performance Training (Power, Precision, and Flow) — 79

What High-Level Function Looks Like at 60+ — 79

Advanced Movement Integration — 83

Practice Plan: Weeks 9–12 — 86

Mental-Physical Synergy — 90

Your Physical Legacy — 93

Chapter 9 — 97

Nutrition and Supplementation for Longevity & Performance	97
Nutrition for Training and Recovery	97
No One-Size-Fits-All: Adapting to Your Diet Philosophy	100
9.4 – Alcohol, Hormones, and Special Considerations	111
Chapter 10	115
Movement Based Arts and Practices	115
Movement Arts as a Lifelong Path	115
Adapting the Practice to Your Season of Life	118
Physical, Mental, and Social Benefits of Practice-Based Movement	121
Walk, Run, Swim, Bicycle	124
Dance	129
Yoga	132
Chapter 11	142
Integration, Adaptation, and Sustained Progress	142
Layering Your Lifestyle	142
Mindset for the Long Haul	145
Linking to Cognitive and Emotional Health	148
Conclusion	151
You're Not Done. You're Just Getting Started.	151
Appendix A	154
References and Resources	154
About the author	158

Chapter 1

A New Model of Fitness for Aging Well

Fit for What?

Let's start with a quiet question.

When you think about being "fit," what comes to mind?

For many of us, especially those of us who grew up on images of cover models and movie stars, fitness has long meant one thing: how you look. Flat stomach. Toned arms. Defined muscles. The kind of body that turns heads at the beach or in a magazine.

But here's the truth—those images were never the full story. And after 50, they stop being useful altogether.

Because the real question isn't *how fit do you look?*

It's *how fit are you for the life you want to live?*

Can you lift your groceries without strain? Can you catch your balance if you trip on a curb? Can you walk for an hour without tiring—or get up from the floor without help? These are the kinds of questions that actually matter. Not just to your safety, but to your freedom.

So let's redefine fitness. Let's talk about strength—not to impress, but to protect. Let's talk about balance—not just on one foot, but in your whole body and life. Let's talk about endurance, recovery, and resilience. These aren't buzzwords. They're the true foundation of aging well.

In the coming pages, we'll look at what the science actually says about staying strong and mobile as we get older. Here's a hint: it has little to do with six-packs and everything to do with something called VO_2 max, which measures how efficiently your body uses oxygen. Or your grip strength, which research shows can predict longevity better than cholesterol. Or your power—the ability to move quickly and with control—which becomes even more important than raw strength after 60.

This book isn't about chasing youth.

It's about training for capability—for the life you still want to live.

And it's about doing that with intelligence, intention, and compassion for yourself. Because wherever you are today, you can build from here. You are not too late. You are not behind.

You're just beginning a different kind of journey. One based not on image, but on capacity.

And the rewards are far greater than a number on the scale.

They're measured in confidence. In freedom. In knowing your body still belongs to you—and will keep showing up for the things that matter most.

Let's begin.

CHAPTER 1

The Longevity Triad

If there's one secret to aging well—not just adding years, but adding *good* years—it's this: train what matters most.

Science has made it abundantly clear that three factors above all others predict how well you'll move, feel, and function as you age. Not cholesterol. Not weight. Not how flexible you are in yoga class.

The big three?

Muscle mass. VO_2 max. Mobility.

Together, they form what we call the Longevity Triad—a simple but powerful framework for training your future self.

Muscle mass isn't just about strength—it's about survival. As we age, we naturally lose muscle unless we train to keep it. That loss, called sarcopenia, quietly robs us of energy, balance, and independence. But it's also reversible. Strength training—even in small doses—can rebuild what time tries to take away.

VO_2 max is your body's capacity to use oxygen. Think of it as your cardiovascular horsepower. It's the single strongest predictor of all-cause mortality. In plain English: the better your VO_2 max, the longer—and better—you're likely to live. And here's the good news: it's remarkably trainable, even in your 60s, 70s, or beyond.

Mobility is your ability to move freely and with control. Not just touching your toes, but standing up from a chair, twisting to reach a high shelf, or stepping over a puddle. It's part balance, part flexibility, part coordination—and it's a make-or-break skill for living independently.

So when does decline begin? For most people, it's surprisingly early—late 30s or early 40s. But that decline is gradual at first. And more importantly, it's not destiny. With consistent training, you can slow, stop, or even reverse much of it.

This is why benchmarks matter. Knowing where you stand—not compared to others, but compared to where you *want* to be—gives you a roadmap.

In your 50s, the focus might be preserving muscle and building aerobic capacity.

In your 60s, it might shift to power (how quickly you can move), agility, and preventing falls.

In your 70s and beyond, the emphasis becomes maintaining what you've built—staying mobile, strong, and confident in your movements.

Wherever you are now, the next step isn't a mystery.

It's measurable. It's trainable. And it's yours to take.

You don't have to do it all at once. You don't even have to do it perfectly.

But you do have to begin.

Because the choices you make now shape the years ahead—not just how long you live, but *how well.*

Training to Stay Capable

Here's the truth no one told most of us in our youth: after 50, movement is no longer optional.

That doesn't mean you have to hit the gym seven days a week or sign up for marathons. But it *does* mean this: if you want to stay strong, mobile, and independent into your later decades, you have to train for it. Not just hope for it.

Why?

Because the body adapts to whatever you ask of it—or don't. If you challenge it with movement, it grows stronger, more capable, more resilient. If you don't... it quietly begins to fade.

And not just strength. We're talking balance. Reaction time. Bone density. The ability to catch yourself from a fall or lift a suitcase overhead without strain. These are the invisible threads that hold your freedom together.

That's why we don't just talk about "working out" in this book. We talk about training.

Training is deliberate. It's specific. And it's designed to build your capacity, not just burn calories.

Think of it in three layers:

Daily activity is your baseline. Walking the dog. Taking the stairs. Gardening. Moving through your day with intention. This is the "movement nutrition" your body needs just to stay well.

Exercise is what most people think of—classes, cardio sessions, yoga, a swim. It raises your heart rate, gets you sweaty, and helps maintain health.

Training goes a step further. It's structured. It has a purpose. It targets a specific outcome—like improving your VO_2 max, building leg strength, or regaining shoulder mobility. It's not about intensity—it's about direction.

All three layers matter. But after 50, the training layer becomes essential. Because without it, we don't just stagnate—we decline.

Think of your future self as someone you care about deeply. What would you want to hand them?

Strong legs to climb stairs? A steady core to prevent falls? The ability to get up from the floor without struggle? That version of you is built now, not later.

Every rep, every walk, every mobility drill is a deposit into the bank account of your future strength.

And the best part?
It's never too late to start.

The Mind-Body Loop

Here's something powerful—and maybe even life-changing—to understand about fitness after 50:

You're not just training your body.

You're training your brain.

Every time you move with intention, every time you breathe through a challenge, every time you show up and do the work—you're rewiring your mind. You're not just lifting weights or walking laps. You're building clarity. Stability. Focus. Mood.

This is the mind-body loop in action. And it's not philosophy—it's neuroscience.

Physical training activates parts of the brain tied to executive function: decision-making, focus, emotional regulation. It boosts neuroplasticity—the brain's ability to adapt, grow, and form new connections. Movement, especially when it's coordinated and purposeful, turns on networks that help you think better, remember more, and stay emotionally balanced.

And the chemistry? It's better than any supplement.

Exercise releases **dopamine** (for motivation and reward), **serotonin** (for calm and mood balance), and **endorphins** (for pain relief and euphoria). These are your natural antidepressants, your built-in energizers. They don't just make you feel better after you work out—they make it easier to want to keep going.

But here's something even more surprising: your *attitude* while you train changes the outcome.

This is called the placebo—or more accurately, the *expectation* effect. If you believe your training will make you stronger, sharper, and more capable… your brain actually helps make that true. It releases different signals. It adjusts effort. It builds in anticipation of success.

That's not wishful thinking. That's real biology.

And when you add **cognitive engagement**—focusing your attention during exercise, tuning into how your body moves, performing reps with intention—you multiply the impact.

We call this the mind-muscle connection. Martial artists know it. Dancers live by it. Neuroscience now confirms it.

So don't just go through the motions. Don't tune out while you move. Tune in.

Bring your full self—mind and body—into the practice.

Because when you do, something extraordinary happens.

You stop just exercising.

You start transforming.

Science Snapshot: Key Takeaways from Chapter 1

- **Muscle Mass Predicts Longevity:** Research shows that low muscle mass is linked to higher mortality, especially in older adults. Resistance training helps reverse age-related sarcopenia and reduces fall risk and frailty.*[Source: "Sarcopenia: European consensus on definition and diagnosis", Age and Ageing, 2010]*
- **VO_2 Max Is the #1 Predictor of All-Cause Mortality:** Just moving from a "low" VO_2 max to "below average" can cut mortality risk by over 50%. VO_2 max is trainable at any age with consistent aerobic conditioning.*[Source: Blair SN,*

et al. "Influence of physical fitness and other precursors on cardiovascular disease and all-cause mortality in men and women." JAMA, 1996]
- **Mobility Decline Begins in Midlife:** Loss of mobility can start subtly in the 40s and 50s but accelerates without intervention. Targeted training can maintain and even improve joint function and movement quality.[Source: Hicks GE, et al. "Mobility and its correlates in older adults", Journal of Aging and Health, 2012]
- **Training vs. Exercise:** Daily movement and casual workouts are great—but training involves progressive overload and specific goals. It's the only method shown to consistently improve functional capacity in aging bodies.[Source: Peterson MD, et al. "Resistance exercise for muscular strength in older adults: a meta-analysis", Ageing Research Reviews, 2010]
- **Exercise Improves Brain Health:** Regular physical training increases hippocampal volume, enhances executive function, and supports emotional regulation.[Source: Erickson KI, et al. "Exercise training increases size of hippocampus and improves memory", PNAS, 2011]
- **Your Attitude Matters:** Studies show that belief in the benefits of exercise can enhance results—even changing biomarkers like cortisol and blood pressure through expectancy effects.[Source: Crum AJ & Langer EJ, "Mind-set matters: Exercise and the placebo effect", Psychological Science, 2007]
- **Cognitive Engagement Multiplies Impact:** Focusing mentally during exercise—counting reps, visualizing movements, correcting form—activates more brain regions and enhances motor learning.[Source: Taubert M, et al. "Dynamic

properties of human brain structure: learning-related changes in cortical areas and associated fiber connections", The Journal of Neuroscience, 2010]

Chapter 2

The Fundamentals of a Fit Life

Move Every Day (Baseline Movement Habits)

Let's begin with something simple. Not flashy, not strenuous—just powerful:
Move your body, every day.

It doesn't have to be a workout. It doesn't even have to break a sweat. But after 50, your body craves daily motion like a plant craves sunlight. Without it, things stiffen. Energy drops. Joints start whispering—or shouting. And the longer you stay still, the harder it is to get going again.

This is where the magic of **NEAT** comes in—short for *Non-Exercise Activity Thermogenesis*. It's a fancy term for the movement you do when you're not "exercising." Walking to the mailbox. Stretching while you wait for coffee. Reaching, squatting, carrying, standing.

These small, simple motions add up in a big way.

In fact, NEAT may play a larger role in your daily energy expenditure—and your long-term vitality—than the workouts you plan. And the best part? It's easy to fit into real life.

Start by breaking the **sedentary cycle**. If you sit for long periods (and most of us do), try a posture reset every 30–60 minutes. Stand up. Roll your shoulders. Twist gently side to side. Take a short walk down the hall or outside.

Think of these as "mobility snacks." They don't take long, but they nourish your joints and wake up your muscles.

Walking is your secret weapon. It's accessible, low-impact, and wildly underrated. A brisk 10-minute walk can improve blood sugar, reduce inflammation, and even brighten your mood. Three walks a day? That's a baseline fitness habit.

Movement doesn't need to be scheduled—it just needs to be frequent. Instead of "fitting in" fitness, look for ways to build it into your environment:

- Keep light weights or a resistance band near your desk.
- Do calf raises while brushing your teeth.
- Put on music and stretch or dance for five minutes before dinner.

These aren't just tricks. They're lifelines.

Because the real goal here isn't to burn calories—it's to **stay alive in your body**. To keep your systems humming. To feel connected, capable, and awake.

Daily movement is the foundation on which everything else is built.

And it's the first promise you can make to yourself:

I will move today.

Even a little. Especially when I don't feel like it.

Because movement is how I say yes to life.

Build and Keep Muscle (Strength & Resistance)

Muscle isn't just about looking fit. It's about staying alive and independent.

After 50, something subtle—but significant—starts to happen. Your body begins to lose muscle mass each year, even if your weight stays the same. This process is called **sarcopenia**, and left unchecked, it accelerates with age.

But here's the powerful part: you can stop it. You can even reverse it.

Muscle is one of the most trainable tissues in the human body. With consistent resistance work, you can build strength well into your 70s, 80s, and beyond.

And this isn't just about lifting weights in a gym. It's about being strong enough to carry groceries. To climb stairs. To rise from the floor without needing help. To brace yourself during a stumble and stay upright.

In this way, **strength is survival**. It's what keeps you autonomous. Capable. In control of your life.

Building muscle also has ripple effects. It improves insulin sensitivity, supports bone density, reduces inflammation, and even boosts mood through powerful hormonal shifts.

So how do you build and keep it?

The key is **resistance**—applying force against your muscles so they adapt and grow stronger. If you enjoy it, you can join a gym or club but you certainly can build muscle with doing so. You don't need fancy equipment. What you need is intention, consistency, and just enough challenge to spark change.

Here are a few accessible options:

- **Bodyweight exercises:** squats, pushups (even against a

wall), step-ups, planks.
- **Resistance bands:** portable, affordable, and great for joint-friendly strength work.
- **Dumbbells or kettlebells:** perfect for home routines—start light and build slowly.
- **Gym-based machines or free weights:** excellent for targeting specific muscle groups with support.

Start where you are. Modify as needed. And remember: proper form and gradual progression matter more than speed or load.

The goal isn't to impress anyone.

It's to stay ready for the life you want to live.

Train your muscles like your future depends on them.

Because it does.

Breathe, Push, Recover (Cardio and Conditioning)

Your heart is more than a muscle. It's your engine.

And how well it pumps, how efficiently it delivers oxygen to your body—that single factor, known as **VO_2 max**, is one of the strongest predictors of your overall health and longevity.

In simple terms, VO_2 max is how well your body uses oxygen during exertion. The higher it is, the more capacity you have to live, move, recover, and respond to life's physical demands.

And here's the best part: it's trainable. At any age.

Even modest improvements in VO_2 max—especially after 50—are linked to longer lifespan and greater vitality.

So how do we train it?

Through **cardiovascular conditioning**—but with strategy, not guesswork. Two approaches are especially effective, and both have a place in a balanced plan:

Zone 2 Cardio

This is steady, moderate effort. You can talk, but singing would be hard. Walking briskly, cycling at a smooth pace, or light jogging are common examples.

Zone 2 builds your aerobic base. It improves mitochondrial function, lowers resting heart rate, and builds endurance without overstressing your system. It's gentle but powerful—especially over time.

High-Intensity Interval Training (HIIT)

HIIT alternates short bursts of high effort with periods of rest or lighter movement. Think: 30 seconds of fast pedaling followed by 90 seconds of easy cycling. Or bodyweight intervals—squats, step-ups, or marching in place.

HIIT trains your heart to respond quickly and recover efficiently. It raises VO_2 max fast—but it's more taxing, so it should be used sparingly and wisely, especially if you're new to training.

The Balance: Push, Then Recover

Too much intensity with too little recovery can backfire, leading to fatigue, poor sleep, or even injury. On the other hand, too little effort means you won't see progress.

The sweet spot? A mix.

- Two to three Zone 2 sessions per week
- One optional HIIT session if appropriate
- Movement every day, even light walking or stretching

And always: rest and **recovery** as part of the plan, not afterthoughts.

You don't need to punish yourself to get results.

You just need to breathe, move with purpose, and give your body what it needs to come back stronger.

This is how you train your engine.

This is how you keep going.

Balance, Mobility, and Joint Care

Let's talk about something no one wants to think about—but everyone over 50 needs to: falling.

Falls are the leading cause of injury in older adults. But here's the hopeful truth: most falls are *preventable.* They're not random. They're the result of systems—balance, joint control, coordination—being neglected until they falter.

But just like muscle and cardio capacity, balance and mobility are trainable.

You can rebuild what time has started to take. You can improve your confidence with every step. You can move through the world not with fear—but with quiet control.

Balance isn't just a single skill—it's an orchestra of inputs: inner ear, vision, muscle strength, and brain coordination. When one system weakens, the others work harder. That's why a holistic approach works best.

Start with Slow Movement

Practices like **Tai Chi** or slow martial arts forms teach you to move with intention, awareness, and control. These arts are centuries old because they work. They train you to center your weight, engage your core, and stay mentally present with every shift and step.

You don't have to learn a full form to benefit. Even standing on one leg while brushing your teeth, or slowly rising from a seated position without using your hands, builds balance.

Add Joint Prep and Mobility

Your joints crave attention. Without regular movement through their full range, they stiffen. And stiff joints can't respond quickly when you trip, reach, or twist.

Daily **joint prep** routines—like slow circles with the ankles, hips, and shoulders—keep tissues supple and signal your brain that these ranges are safe.

Mobility is more than flexibility. It's the ability to control motion. To move smoothly and with strength through every angle your life might require.

Make It a Ritual

Balance and mobility don't need to be an extra workout. They can be woven into your day like breath.

- Ankle rolls while waiting for the kettle
- Controlled step-ups on the stairs
- Hip circles or gentle squats during TV breaks
- A few minutes of Tai Chi-inspired movement each morning

These small rituals become anchors. They remind your body how to move well—and your mind that you're not fragile.

You are capable. You are improving. You are building a body that trusts itself.

Recovery as Training

Here's a mindset shift that changes everything:

Recovery isn't what you do after the real work. It *is* the work.

Especially after 50, recovery isn't just helpful—it's vital. Your body repairs, rebuilds, and upgrades itself when you rest—not while you're lifting weights or running laps. Training without recovery is just wearing yourself down.

Think of it this way: every workout is a *withdrawal* from your energy account. Recovery is the *deposit* that makes future effort possible. If you keep withdrawing without putting anything back, eventually, you go into deficit—physically, mentally, and emotionally.

So what fuels that recovery account?

The Big Three: Sleep, Downtime, and Protein

- **Sleep** is your #1 recovery tool. During deep sleep, your body repairs tissues, balances hormones, and clears out inflammation. Aim for 7–9 hours, and don't underestimate the power of naps.
- **Downtime** matters too. This isn't laziness—it's strategic rest. Quiet walks. Gentle stretching. Time outdoors. Anything that brings your nervous system out of stress mode and into repair mode.
- **Protein** provides the raw materials for muscle repair and immune support. After 50, your body becomes less efficient at using protein, so it becomes even more important to get enough—ideally spread across meals.

Your Body Talks—Learn to Listen

Technology like **heart rate variability (HRV)** trackers can offer insights into how recovered you are. Low HRV, persistent fatigue, or unusual soreness can be signs you're pushing too hard or not recovering enough.

You don't need fancy devices to pay attention. Simple signs matter:

- Do you feel energized or drained after training?
- Are you sleeping well?
- Is your motivation dipping without clear cause?

Recovery is about rhythm. It's about *responding* to your body, not overriding it.

The Recovery Bank

After 50, your recovery "interest rate" changes. It takes longer to bounce back, and the margin for error narrows. But that's not a problem—it's an opportunity.

With consistency, you can build up a **Recovery Bank** that protects your energy, preserves your enthusiasm, and keeps progress going strong.

Every good night's sleep, every rest day honored, every protein-rich meal is a deposit.

You're not being soft. You're being smart.

And smart training means knowing when to push—and when to pause.

Because your next level of strength is waiting.

It just needs the right space to grow.

Work/Recovery Balance Checklist

Use this weekly check-in to stay in rhythm—not just with your workouts, but with your *recovery*, too.

Work (Effort & Challenge)

- I moved with purpose at least 5 days this week.
- I completed at least 2 strength or resistance sessions.
- I trained my cardiovascular system (Zone 2 or intervals) at least 2 times.
- I practiced at least one balance or mobility-focused activity.

- I had moments of challenge that made me breathe harder, focus deeper, or feel alive.

Recovery (Repair & Recharge)

- I got at least 7 hours of sleep most nights.
- I had at least one full day of active recovery or rest.
- I ate enough protein to support my training and healing.
- I felt generally energized—not chronically tired or sore.
- I took time to breathe, stretch, or reflect in a quiet space.

Overall Rhythm

- I felt balanced between effort and ease.
- I listened to my body and adjusted when needed.
- I felt proud of showing up—for both the work and the rest.

If you checked most boxes on both sides, you're training wisely and sustainably. If recovery is lagging—start there. That's where your next breakthrough begins.

Chapter 3

The Psychology of Lifelong Fitness

The Identity Shift

Let's be honest—most of us didn't grow up thinking of ourselves as "athletes." Especially if fitness was something we came to later in life, or if we've had long stretches of inactivity, illness, or simply other priorities.

So it's natural to carry around quiet doubts:

"I'm too old for this."

"I've never been a workout person."

"I just don't have that kind of body."

But what if none of that has to define you anymore?

What if the real shift isn't in your body—but in your identity?

Because here's something powerful: **identity drives behavior.** When you see yourself as "someone who trains," your actions begin to align with that story. You don't have to be perfect. You just have to show up from that place.

You're not training to impress anyone. You're training because you've decided to live fully, to take responsibility for your strength and capacity. That decision doesn't belong to the young. It belongs to *you*.

And that means:

- You're not "too old." You're *not done*.
- You're not trying to "get back" to anything. You're building forward.
- You don't have to look a certain way. You just have to *move like someone who matters*.

When you train, you're not just shaping muscles. You're reshaping your story. You're becoming someone who responds to challenge with courage. Someone who chooses action over decline. Someone who claims their body as a living, evolving part of who they are—not just who they were.

And you don't need anyone's permission to claim that.

Let fitness become part of your identity—not as a job, or a punishment, or a "should," but as a gift you give yourself.

Because the moment you say, *"This is who I am now"*—you open a door that can never close.

You're not aiming to become someone else.

You're returning to your strength.

Motivation, Meaning, and Momentum

There's nothing wrong with wanting to look good.

But here's the truth: *aesthetics alone won't carry you through the long haul.*

Because the moment things get tough—the weather's bad, the schedule's packed, the knees are sore—*vanity fades.* It doesn't reach deep enough.

What does?

Meaning.

When you train to look a certain way, you're borrowing motivation. When you train to *live* a certain way, you're building it from within.

This is the heart of **intrinsic motivation**—the kind that lasts. You're not working out because someone told you to, or because of guilt, or to chase a number on the scale. You're moving because movement protects your lifestyle. Because it lets you pick up your grandchild. Hike that trail. Sleep through the night. Stay sharp and steady and sovereign in your own body.

That kind of meaning has gravity.

And when fitness becomes *something you don't want to lose*—momentum builds. You stop seeing it as a task and start treating it like a privilege. A quiet, daily act of devotion to your future self.

So how do you find that kind of motivation?

Ask yourself:

- What kind of life do I want ten years from now?
- What am I afraid of losing—and how can training help me keep it?
- Who benefits when I take care of myself?

This isn't about pressure. It's about clarity.

When you know your *why*, you stop starting over. You stop arguing with yourself. You just do the work—not perfectly, but consistently—because it matters.

You don't have to be motivated every day.

You just have to know what's at stake.

And once you feel the joy of momentum—the quiet pride of being someone who *does* what they said they would—you start to move not from willpower, but from identity.

And that's when everything changes.

Habit Stacking and Environmental Design

Motivation is powerful—but it's also unpredictable.

Some days, it's there when you wake up. Other days… not so much.

That's why sustainable fitness doesn't rely on willpower.

It relies on **structure.**

And one of the most effective ways to create structure is by shaping your environment—so that movement becomes not a decision you have to wrestle with, but the *default setting* of your day.

Start with Strategic Triggers

Your brain loves patterns. When one thing happens, it expects the next thing. You can use this to your advantage by **stacking habits**—pairing a new action with something you already do.

- After I brush my teeth, I do 10 calf raises.
- While the coffee brews, I stretch my shoulders.
- After I check the mail, I take a five-minute walk around the block.

These aren't workouts. They're anchors. And they build momentum without friction.

Use Wearable Cues and Reminders

Visual and tactile cues help keep your goals top of mind. Lay out your workout clothes the night before. Keep a resistance band near your desk. Set a recurring calendar nudge or alarm labeled with your "why."

And if you wear a tracker or smartwatch? Let it be a gentle partner—not a pressure device. Use it to celebrate consistency, not chase perfection.

Build in Social Accountability

We're more likely to follow through when someone else knows we're trying. You don't need a workout buddy every day—but telling a friend your goal, sharing your progress, or joining a challenge group can be a game-changer.

And if you're not "social"? No problem. Even a quiet checkmark on a wall calendar can offer the same kind of feedback loop.

Create a Frictionless Environment

Make the healthy choice the easy one.

- Clear a small space where you can move freely.
- Keep light equipment visible and ready.
- Put a yoga mat or towel somewhere you'll trip over it—in the best way.

When fitness is woven into your environment, it stops being an interruption. It becomes part of how you live.

And that's the goal: **not a program you start and stop, but a life you build and sustain.**

Because when your environment supports your identity, everything becomes just a little bit easier.

And easier means more likely.

And more likely means lasting.

Chapter 4

The ACF Model – High-Functioning Movement After 50

What Is ACF?

Let's start with a simple idea that can quietly transform how you think about fitness after 50:

You're not here to *maintain* yourself.

You're here to *grow*.

For most of modern history, the story we've been told about aging is that it's about decline. That the best you can do is hold on to what you have—slow the losses, manage the inevitable slide. But this mindset misses something profound:

Your body—and your mind—are built for adaptation. Even now. Especially now.

That's where ACF comes in.

Applied Cognitive Fitness isn't just a system. It's a way of living. A set of principles born from decades of real-world experience—training, teaching, creating, and staying curious. It's about harnessing the synergy between movement and thought, effort and reflection, challenge and purpose.

ACF was shaped by a lifetime spent doing things most people said couldn't—or shouldn't—be done past a certain age: composing music, performing, studying martial arts, teaching, writing, flying, learning new technology. The pattern that emerged was clear: the people who stayed engaged, who kept learning and moving with intention, didn't just *maintain.* They evolved.

This model is built on one radical belief:

Growth is possible at any age.

Not only that—it can be richer, more rewarding, and more meaningful precisely because of everything you've already lived.

That's why in this book, ACF isn't just about cognitive improvement in the abstract. It's about how your brain and your body work together to create a life you actually want to live.

Because movement is never just movement. Every time you lift, balance, step, or stretch, you're also training:

- Attention
- Coordination
- Pattern recognition
- Emotional regulation
- Decision-making under pressure

You're teaching your nervous system to stay adaptable. You're creating a brain that doesn't just *remember* but *responds.*

That's the essence of cognitive-physical synergy—the idea that when you train your body with intention, you're also building a more capable, resilient mind.

And here's the most hopeful part: this isn't a theory. It's reality. From martial artists in their 70s to lifelong dancers, from pilots to teachers, the same pattern shows up again and again: your systems can keep improving if you give them the right inputs—challenge, purpose, consistency, and recovery.

In the next sections, you'll explore the seven core principles of ACF, see how they apply to physical vitality, and learn how to put them into practice in a way that feels authentic, sustainable, and alive.

Because you're not done.

You're just entering a new stage of possibility.

The 7 ACF Principles Applied to Physical Vitality

Before we dive into each principle, let's step back and look at where ACF comes from.

Applied Cognitive Fitness (ACF) is a framework I developed over decades of living, teaching, creating, and staying curious. It grew out of a question that kept coming up again and again:

What if getting older doesn't have to mean getting worse?

In the mental realm, research increasingly shows that some abilities can *improve* with age—especially when we stay engaged in meaningful, challenging activities. Many of the techniques in ACF are drawn from neuroscience, psychology, and learning science. They've been proven to help preserve and even grow capacities like memory, focus, pattern recognition, and emotional regulation—well into later life.

This is the heart of ACF:

A belief that growth is possible at any age—if you approach it with purpose, strategy, and engagement.

In the cognitive domain, this means:

- Learning new skills, not just maintaining old ones
- Practicing retrieval, not just passive review
- Staying emotionally invested, not just going through motions
- Embracing challenge as fuel for adaptation

Over time, I began to notice how these same principles could also be applied to physical training—because the body and brain are inseparable. Movement is never only mechanical. It's also cognitive and emotional. The nervous system doesn't distinguish between "mental practice" and "physical practice." It simply responds to signals.

But here's where we need to be clear:

While the mind can continue expanding in some ways indefinitely, the body does have limits. Biology matters. Muscle mass, bone density, reaction time—they can all be improved, but never indefinitely. That's not a flaw—it's simply the reality of being human. Even the most gifted athletes eventually retire, not because they stop caring or trying, but because no system can grow forever.

So in this book, ACF is not presented as a miracle cure. It's a set of powerful tools that can help you get the most from your training, sustain your motivation, and deepen your connection to movement. But it's only one part of the bigger picture—alongside smart programming, recovery, and respect for the body's changing needs.

If you're curious to explore how ACF applies to mental training in more depth, you'll find other books in this series dedicated to that. For now, let's look at how each principle can help you move with more purpose, awareness, and vitality.

1. Use It to Improve It

In the cognitive realm:

Your brain is like a living network. The pathways you use most become stronger. When you recall names, practice languages, or solve problems, you're strengthening those circuits.

Applied to the body:

Muscles, bones, and connective tissue respond the same way. Use them, and they adapt. Stop using them, and they weaken. This is why consistent movement matters more than heroic effort. A little bit, done regularly, preserves capacity.

The principle is simple: *Whatever you hope to keep or improve—use it often.*

2. Learn What Matters

In the cognitive realm:

ACF encourages learning things that are meaningful and relevant to you. The brain retains best what it cares about. Abstract drills fade; purpose-driven learning sticks.

Applied to the body:

It's the same with training. You're more likely to stay engaged when you focus on movement that improves *your* life—whether that's getting off the floor easily, hiking with friends, or feeling steady on uneven ground.

Ask yourself: *What movements matter most to my real-world freedom?* Start there.

3. Train with Purpose

In the cognitive realm:

Mindless repetition doesn't grow capacity. Purposeful, goal-oriented practice does. ACF emphasizes setting intentions for each session.

Applied to the body:

Don't just show up to "get it over with." Show up to build something—strength, balance, resilience. Even if it's only ten minutes, bring intention to it.

Training with purpose helps you notice progress and stay motivated when the novelty wears off.

4. Limit Passive Input

In the cognitive realm:

We live in an era of distraction. Divided attention weakens learning. ACF encourages limiting passive consumption and practicing focus.

Applied to the body:

This is what I sometimes call the bandwidth paradigm. When you're training with half your attention on your phone, the TV, or your to-do list, you're only getting part of the benefit.

Yes—music can be motivating. Yes—podcasts can pass the time. But at least some of the time, close the extra tabs in your mind. Bring all your attention into the movement itself. Feel your breath, your center of gravity, your muscle engagement.

Dancers, yogis, martial artists—this is their secret. They train the nervous system through presence. That's where real change happens.

5. Focus on Output

In the cognitive realm:

Passive reading or listening doesn't wire the brain the way active output does. Retrieval, creation, and teaching lock knowledge in place.

Applied to the body:

In movement, output means action. Doing the reps. Testing

your balance. Practicing under mild pressure.

Thinking about fitness doesn't build fitness. You have to *express* what you're learning.

6. Live with Stakes

In the cognitive realm:

When learning matters to you—emotionally, socially, practically—it sticks. Stakes create urgency and purpose.

Applied to the body:

Physical training becomes non-optional when you connect it to something real. Protecting your independence. Avoiding preventable injuries. Staying ready for the moments that matter.

Remind yourself: *This isn't just exercise. This is preparation for the life I want to keep living.*

7. Perform Better Than You Practice

In the cognitive realm:

ACF teaches that when you practice consistently, your performance often exceeds your expectations—especially under real-world conditions.

Applied to the body:

When you train balance, strength, and mobility with presence and intention, you'll be amazed how your body shows up for you when you need it.

The slip you recover from.

The load you can lift without strain.

The energy you didn't realize you had.

This is the hidden promise of steady, mindful practice.

ACF is not a magic wand.

It won't stop the clock or make you invulnerable. But it *will* help you reclaim more of what's possible—by aligning your attention, intention, and effort.

Because your body is still capable of growth.

And your mind is still capable of guiding it.

The ACF Pyramid Applied to Movement

If ACF has a visual symbol, it's a pyramid.

Think of it like this:

- The base is what you do consistently—your everyday movement, mindset, and recovery.
- The middle is how you progressively challenge yourself.
- The top is the performance that emerges when the other layers are in place.

In the cognitive realm, this model shows how learning builds: you start with frequent exposure, add progressively harder challenges, and finally demonstrate mastery under real conditions.

Applied to movement, the pyramid helps you balance four elements: load, challenge zones, recovery, and performance.

Let's look at each one:

Load

Load simply means the amount of stress or demand you place on your body.

This could be:

- The weight you lift

- The speed you walk
- The time you hold a position
- The complexity of a movement

Load is necessary. Without it, your muscles and nervous system don't get the signal to adapt. But more isn't always better. Load must be appropriate to your current capacity—and adjusted gradually.

Think of it like adding weight to a barbell. Too little, and nothing changes. Too much, and you risk injury. Just enough, and you grow.

Challenge Zones

Once you establish a baseline of load, you expand into challenge zones.

These are deliberate forays beyond your comfort level—moments when your body and mind have to work a little harder:

- A slightly heavier weight
- A longer duration
- A more unstable surface
- A faster pace

Challenge zones are where adaptation happens. They should feel uncomfortable—but not overwhelming.

This is why presence matters. You need enough focus to sense the difference between *good challenge* and *danger*.

If you can talk easily through a movement, you're probably not challenging yourself. If you feel panic or pain, you've overshot the mark.

Aim for the space in between—where you're working, but

still in control.

Recovery

If challenge is the accelerator, recovery is the brake—and you need both.

Recovery isn't passive laziness. It's active repair. It's when your muscles rebuild, your nervous system recalibrates, and your reserves refill.

Recovery can look like:

- Sleep
- Gentle movement
- Hydration and nutrition
- Breathing practices
- Time in nature
- Mental disengagement from training

In ACF, recovery is not an afterthought. It's planned as intentionally as load and challenge.

After 50, the recovery phase often needs more attention. Respect that. You're not "falling behind." You're training wisely.

Performance

When you balance load, challenge, and recovery consistently, you unlock better performance.

Performance doesn't mean winning medals or setting records. It means:

- Feeling stronger in daily life
- Recovering faster from effort

- Moving with more confidence and less pain
- Responding to real-world demands with grace and power

This is the top of the pyramid. It's not something you "achieve" once. It's something you experience again and again in small, satisfying ways:

- The day you notice you carried groceries without strain
- The walk that feels easier than it used to
- The moment you catch your balance without thinking

That's your training showing up for you.

Balancing Stress and Repair
Here's the simplest way to remember this model:
Stress + Recovery = Growth.
Too much stress without recovery leads to breakdown.
Too little stress, even with perfect recovery, leads to stagnation.
The sweet spot is a dynamic rhythm between the two.
You don't have to get it perfect. You just have to pay attention.
Listen to your body.
Respect your limits.
Test them, gently.
Then give yourself the space to rebuild.
That's how you move from maintenance to improvement.
That's how you build a body—and a mindset—ready for the next chapter.

Life as Training: A Story-Based Overview

It's one thing to read about principles like "Use It to Improve It" or "Train With Purpose." It's another to see them in action.

So let me share a little of what this has looked like in my own life—not because you need to do any of the same things, but because these stories show what's possible when you treat life itself as your training ground.

I didn't grow up imagining I'd someday write books about movement or cognition. But looking back, I can see a clear pattern: a commitment to learning, to showing up when it mattered, and to using every experience as a chance to build something new—inside myself.

The Musician's Mindset

From the time I was very young, music demanded both skill and presence. In a performance, there was nowhere to hide. You prepared, you rehearsed, and then—no matter how you felt—you stepped onto the stage.

Music taught me that practice is not the same as performance—and that the gap between them can shrink with deliberate training. When the adrenaline came, I learned to welcome it. To breathe, smile, and engage.

This experience became the foundation for one of my most powerful beliefs:

You can perform better than you practice—if you respect the process.

The Martial Artist's Body

Years later, I found martial arts—another path that merged physical discipline with mental clarity.

In the dojo, you don't just train your body. You train your awareness. You learn to feel where your weight is centered, to track subtle shifts in an opponent, to stay calm when your heart is racing.

Martial arts taught me about the bandwidth paradigm—the difference between moving automatically and moving with full engagement. When you close the mental tabs and give your attention fully to the moment, your body responds differently.

Balance improves. Timing sharpens. You discover reserves of energy you didn't know you had.

The Paramedic's Stakes

Some lessons came from places where the stakes were higher—where mistakes could carry real consequences.

When I trained as a paramedic in my 40s, the learning curve was steep. Lives depended on getting it right. In those situations, theory alone wasn't enough. You had to stay calm, make decisions, and trust your training under pressure.

That's where the ACF principle Live With Stakes took on new meaning. When the outcomes matter deeply, your brain pays attention in a different way. Stress becomes a sharpening force instead of a blunting one.

This is why I often say that purposeful training—especially when connected to real consequence—builds a different kind of capacity.

The Pilot's Clarity

Earning my pilot's license in my 50s added another layer: the discipline of checklists, the rigor of preparation, and the calm required to handle complexity.

Flying isn't about reacting emotionally. It's about responding with clarity. That mindset applies to everything—fitness included.

You prepare your body. You prepare your mind. And then you trust that preparation when it counts.

The Teacher's Integration

Teaching martial arts and music pulled it all together. When you teach, you see your own patterns more clearly. You learn to explain what once felt instinctive. You become accountable not just to yourself, but to your students.

Teaching is the ultimate output.

It forces you to keep learning. It challenges you to embody what you share.

The Thread That Connects It All

Across these experiences, one truth kept surfacing:

Life is the best training ground you'll ever have.

You don't have to become a performer, a martial artist, or a pilot. But you *can* decide to approach your own movement practice—and your own learning—with that same spirit of engagement.

Show up with purpose.

Connect your effort to something that matters.

Let the stakes sharpen your focus.

And know that every moment of practice—whether in a gym, a living room, or simply walking outside—is part of a much bigger story.

Because in the end, the real goal isn't just to move more easily or to think more clearly.

It's to become someone who keeps growing, no matter what season of life you're in.

Chapter 5

Testing, Tracking, and Personal Metrics

Where Are You Now? The Importance of Baseline Testing

Most of us think we "know" our fitness levels—but without real measurement, we're often guessing. And guesswork doesn't help you build smarter, safer, or more effective training.

That's why we start with **baseline testing**—a snapshot of where your body is today, before you begin transforming it. It's not about labeling yourself, but about illuminating your starting point so you can track real progress.

Why Baseline Testing Matters

1. **Clarity About Your Current Status** Many factors—strength, balance, mobility, cardio capacity—decline as we age, often subtly and quietly. A simple test can reveal hidden weaknesses and give you meaningful insight into your starting point. pliability.com+1sunnyhealthfitness.com +1pmc.ncbi.nlm.nih.govwsj.com+1theguardian.com+1

2. **Personalized Goal Setting** Without knowing your baseline, it's hard to know where you're headed. Baseline metrics help you set realistic, measurable, and motivating goals—whether that's improving your VO$_2$max, increasing your grip strength, or reducing fall risk.
3. **Monitoring Progress Over Time** As you train, periodic retesting lets you see what's improving and what needs more attention. Your plan evolves with your results—not from guesswork.
4. **Safety and Injury Prevention** Testing identifies the areas most in need of support, helping you tune your training to reduce injury risk, especially when strength or balance are limited.

Key Areas to Test

Here are core components to include in a baseline assessment:

- **Strength** (e.g., grip strength test) Grip strength is a simple yet powerful predictor of whole-body function, mortality risk, and cognitive outcomes. myvitalmetrics.com+4sciencedirect.com+4springhills.com+4aarp.org+14pmc.ncbi.nlm.nih.gov+14sciencedirect.com+14
- **Muscle Endurance** (e.g., sit-to-stand or step-up tests) These measure your ability to repeat functional movements. They reflect your readiness for everyday tasks.
- **Balance** (e.g., one-leg stand or timed up-and-go) Poor balance is strongly linked to fall risk. A one-leg stand for 10 seconds, for example, correlates with neuromuscular aging and mortality risk. arxiv.org+7en.wikipedia.org+7arxiv.org+7realsimple.com

- **Mobility** (e.g., reach tests, squat depth, joint range of motion)Improves performance and helps prevent injuries.
- **Cardiovascular Fitness** (e.g., walk-test, step-test, or VO$_2$max estimation)Your VO$_2$max—or its simpler estimate—is among the strongest predictors of all-cause mortality. thesun.co.uk+15healthline.com+15pmc.ncbi.nlm.nih.gov+15

How to Approach Testing

You don't need lab conditions. Most assessments can be done safely at home or in a basic gym setting:

- Use a hand grip dynamometer or a simple squeeze gauge.
- Count how many sit-to-stand repetitions you can do in 30 seconds.
- Time how long you can stand on one leg—ideally 10 seconds or more.
- Track an easy walk test that estimates VO$_2$max using a smartphone app or manual calculation.

This isn't a pass/fail exam—it's information. The goal is not perfection, but insight.

Baseline testing empowers you to train smarter—not harder.

It uncovers your unique profile, invites you to own it, and helps you create a plan that addresses your real strengths and challenges.

When you know where you start, every next step becomes clearer.

And every milestone becomes worth celebrating.

Useful Metrics (and How to Track Them)

Once you've taken your baseline snapshot, the next question is simple:

How do you keep track of your progress?

The good news is, you don't need a lab or expensive equipment to monitor your most important metrics. With just a few simple tests and tools, you can build a clear picture of your evolving capacity—and adjust your training as you go.

These are some of the most useful measures to consider:

Grip Strength
Why it matters:

Grip strength is a surprisingly powerful indicator of overall vitality, predicting not just upper-body strength but also cardiovascular health, cognitive outcomes, and longevity.

How to track it:

- Use a hand dynamometer (affordable handheld devices are available).
- Test every few months.
- Record the highest reading from three attempts on each hand.

Benchmarks:

Average healthy adults 50–70 often see readings from ~20–35 kg (women) and ~35–55 kg (men), but improvement over your own baseline is more important than any chart.

Sit-to-Stand Test
Why it matters:

This test measures lower-body strength and endurance—critical for preventing falls and maintaining independence.

How to track it:

- Sit on a firm chair without armrests.
- Cross your arms over your chest.
- Count how many times you can rise fully to standing and sit again in **30 seconds.**
- Track your score over time.

Benchmark goal:

Most adults over 60 can aim for 12–17 repetitions; fewer than 8 may indicate strength loss.

Step-Up Test

Why it matters:

Step-ups measure leg strength, balance, and aerobic capacity in one simple movement.

How to track it:

- Use an 8–12-inch step or sturdy platform.
- Count how many full step-ups you can complete in 2 minutes at a comfortable, continuous pace.
- Note any instability or fatigue.

Walking Pace and Gait

Why it matters:

Walking speed is often called the "sixth vital sign." It reflects strength, coordination, cardiovascular health, and neurological function.

How to track it:

- Measure how long it takes to walk 4 meters (13 feet).
- A pace slower than 0.8 meters/second (under ~1.8 mph) may indicate increased health risks.
- Pay attention to stride smoothness and symmetry.

Mobility Screens
Why they matter:
Mobility screens help you track flexibility, joint range of motion, and early signs of restriction that could lead to injury.

How to track them:

- Use simple self-checks: overhead reach, ankle dorsiflexion, squat depth, and neck rotation.
- Note any discomfort or limits.
- Repeat every few months to watch for changes.

Pain-Free Range of Motion
Why it matters:
You don't just want movement—you want comfortable movement.

How to track it:

- Use a 0–10 scale (0 = no discomfort, 10 = severe pain).
- Record any areas where pain arises.
- Use this as a guide for gentle mobility work or professional support if needed.

Optional: Wearable Tech and Smart Trackers

Today's devices can offer helpful data, including:

- **Step counts and daily movement** (NEAT)
- **Heart rate variability (HRV)**
- **VO$_2$max estimates**
- **Sleep patterns**
- **Resting heart rate trends**

These tools can be motivating, but remember: **they are tools, not judges.** Their role is to inform your choices, not to define your worth.

How Often Should You Track?

You don't need to obsess over numbers daily. For most people:

- Re-test your strength, mobility, and cardio capacity every **3–4 months.**
- Reassess walking pace and balance **every 6 months.**
- Keep a simple log or journal to see your progress in context.

Progress is rarely linear. You may have plateaus and setbacks. That's normal. What matters most is that you keep showing up—tracking what you can, learning as you go.

Because what gets measured gets managed.

And what gets managed, improves.

Advanced Assessment Tools

Once you've established your baseline and begun tracking your key metrics, you may feel curious about going further.

Advanced assessments can reveal a deeper, more nuanced picture of your body's health and performance. While they're not necessary for everyone, they can be valuable tools—especially if you:

- Want precise measurements to guide your training
- Are coming back from injury or illness
- Need extra motivation to see how training affects your body over time

Here are some of the most useful options:

DEXA Scan
What it measures:

- Bone density (crucial for understanding osteoporosis risk)
- Body composition (lean mass, fat mass, and regional distribution)

Why it matters:
Bone density naturally declines with age, especially after 50. A DEXA scan provides an objective measure so you can monitor and respond proactively.

Where to get it:

- Many hospitals, sports medicine clinics, and imaging centers offer DEXA scanning.

- You don't necessarily need a physician referral, though it can help with insurance coverage.

How often to retest:

- Every 1–2 years if you have low bone density or significant body composition goals.
- Less often if you're primarily tracking trends.

VO_2 Max Testing
What it measures:

- Maximal oxygen uptake—a key indicator of cardiovascular fitness and aerobic capacity.

Why it matters:

VO_2 max is one of the strongest predictors of longevity and overall health. Even modest improvements reduce your risk of chronic disease and mortality.

Ways to test it:

- **Laboratory test:** A treadmill or cycle test with gas analysis is the gold standard for accuracy.
- **Wearable estimates:** Many smartwatches and fitness trackers can approximate VO_2 max using heart rate and pace data. These aren't perfectly precise but are excellent for tracking trends over time.

How often to retest:

- Every 6–12 months.

Resting Metabolic Rate (RMR) Testing
What it measures:

- The number of calories your body burns at rest.
- Helpful if you want to fine-tune nutrition for weight management or energy needs.

Where to get it:

- Many sports performance centers and dietitian offices offer metabolic testing.
- Typically requires fasting for 8–12 hours beforehand.

How often to retest:

- Once or twice a year, or when making significant changes to your training or diet.

Heart Rate Variability (HRV)
What it measures:

- The variation between heartbeats—a sensitive marker of recovery, nervous system balance, and readiness to train.

Why it matters:
Higher HRV generally indicates better recovery and resilience. Chronic low HRV may signal overtraining or high stress.

How to track it:

- Wearable devices (like Oura Ring, Whoop, Garmin, and Polar) measure HRV passively while you sleep.
- Some apps can record HRV in the morning using a chest strap.

How often to track:

- Daily tracking gives the clearest trend over time.
- Focus on averages and patterns rather than day-to-day fluctuations.

Where to Get Tested

Depending on where you live, you'll find these services at:

- Sports medicine clinics
- University research labs
- Medical imaging centers
- Fitness performance facilities
- Some advanced physical therapy practices

If you're unsure where to start, your primary care physician or a reputable personal trainer can help you find resources.

What to Do With the Results

1. **Stay objective.** Numbers are information, not judgment.
2. **Compare to your baseline, not to others.**
3. **Use the data to refine your goals and training plan.**

4. **Retest periodically to measure your progress.**

When Advanced Testing Isn't Necessary

Remember: You don't *have* to pursue advanced assessments to train effectively.

For many people, simple functional tests and consistency are enough. If you enjoy data, great—use it as a tool. But never let it become a burden or a barrier.

The real measure of progress is how you feel, how you function, and how confidently you live in your body.

Summary

Before you start any journey, it helps to know exactly where you stand.

Testing and tracking aren't about judgment or perfection. They're about **clarity.** They give you a real picture of your strengths and your opportunities—and they help you measure progress you might otherwise miss.

Remember:

- **Baseline testing** is your starting line. Simple measures like grip strength, sit-to-stand repetitions, walking speed, and mobility screens reveal where you are right now.
- **Useful metrics** help you stay focused. Regular check-ins on strength, balance, endurance, and range of motion can guide your training decisions and keep you motivated.
- **Advanced assessments**—like DEXA scans, VO_2 max testing, or HRV tracking—are optional tools if you want deeper data. They can be valuable, but they're never required to succeed.

Above all:

Measure what matters to you.

If a number helps you feel inspired, use it.

If a test feels discouraging, reframe it as information, not a verdict.

And always track progress in context—over weeks, months, and years, not days.

Fitness after 50 isn't a pass/fail test. It's a practice of staying engaged, aware, and responsive.

When you take time to learn where you stand, you give yourself the power to train smarter, recover wisely, and celebrate every gain along the way.

Chapter 6

Tier 1: Foundation – Daily Movement

Movement is Non-Negotiable

In this book, you'll see again and again that your fitness isn't built in a single workout, or in a single week.

It's built in layers.

This is why everything here is organized into a **three-tier structure**:

1. **Tier 1:** Daily Movement—the foundation of everything you do.
2. **Tier 2:** Intentional Exercise—structured sessions to build capacity.
3. **Tier 3:** Performance Training—specific challenges to expand your abilities further.

Tier 1—*daily movement*—is where all the other layers sit. It's the soil your strength, endurance, and mobility will grow from.

And that's why we start here.

CHAPTER 6

A Life That Moves

It's easy to think of "fitness" as something separate from the rest of life—a separate appointment, a block of time on your calendar, a box to check so you can feel like you did something good for yourself.

But the truth is: **Your body doesn't separate movement into "exercise" and "everything else."**

Your nervous system and muscles respond to every signal, all day long. Every time you stand up, squat, twist, or walk, you're either reinforcing capacity—or letting it slip away.

And here's the quiet truth: As we get older, the cost of *not moving* grows steeper.

Sitting becomes more than sitting. It becomes tight hips, stiff shoulders, sluggish circulation, slower metabolism, and a creeping sense that you're less capable than you used to be.

But here's the hopeful side of that same truth:

Small movements, repeated consistently, can keep you vibrant.

They remind your body that you still need it.

They tell your muscles, bones, and joints that they still have a job to do.

They keep you in the game.

The Power of NEAT

You'll hear this term a lot: **NEAT**—Non-Exercise Activity Thermogenesis.

It sounds complicated, but it's beautifully simple.

NEAT is everything you do when you're not "working out."

- Getting up to let the dog out.
- Carrying groceries.

- Taking the stairs.
- Gardening.
- Walking across the parking lot.

These ordinary motions can account for more daily movement—and more calorie burn—than your workouts.

More importantly, they keep your joints moving, your blood flowing, and your balance engaged.

If Tier 1 were a sentence, it would be this:

Move more, more often, in more ways.

Why It Matters Now More Than Ever

In our 20s and 30s, we could get away with a lot. A long day on the couch didn't feel like much. A missed workout was easily replaced.

But after 50, the balance tips.

Inactivity doesn't just pause progress.

It begins to quietly subtract from the movement bank you've built up over the years.

And yet—this is exactly why daily movement is so powerful. Because it's simple.

It doesn't require equipment.

It doesn't require perfect health.

It doesn't even require extra time—just different choices.

When you treat movement as non-negotiable—a normal, expected part of your day—something shifts. You stop debating whether you "feel like it." You stop telling yourself you'll start tomorrow.

You just do it—like brushing your teeth or drinking water.

And over time, these moments accumulate into something profound:

CHAPTER 6

A life that keeps moving.

A Quiet Invitation

So consider this your invitation to start where you are:

- If you haven't moved much lately, begin with standing up more often.
- If you're already walking daily, add short bursts of movement every hour.
- If you feel strong, explore new ranges of motion—reaching, squatting, balancing.

You don't have to get it perfect.

You don't have to do it all today.

But you do have to start.

Because daily movement is the baseline of your independence, your energy, and your confidence.

It's the first layer of a body that will keep showing up for you, day after day.

Core Habits for Daily Vitality

Daily movement is more than just a checklist—it's the environment your body lives in.

The beauty of Tier 1 is that it doesn't require dramatic changes. Most of what you need to stay strong and capable is already woven into your day. You just have to learn to see it—and to use it.

When you do, you transform ordinary moments into hidden training.

Posture Resets

One of the simplest—and most powerful—habits you can build is the **posture reset.**

Over time, gravity and habits pull us forward. The head tilts, the shoulders round, the low back stiffens. Left unaddressed, these patterns can turn into pain, limited mobility, and loss of confidence in movement.

But you don't have to accept that as your fate.

A posture reset is a gentle interruption of this drift—a chance to re-stack your spine, open your chest, and reconnect to your breath.

Try this now:

- Stand or sit tall.
- Imagine a string gently lifting the crown of your head.
- Soften your ribs and draw your shoulders back and down.
- Take three slow, deep breaths.

That's it.

One small moment. One signal to your nervous system that you're still awake in your body.

Do this a few times a day—before meals, after phone calls, whenever you remember—and you'll notice how much easier it becomes to stay upright, open, and engaged.

Mobility Snacks

Think of **mobility snacks** as little bites of movement nourishment sprinkled throughout your day.

They don't have to be long or complicated. Just short, intentional motions that keep your joints supple and your muscles switched on:

- Ankle circles while brushing your teeth.
- Shoulder rolls while waiting for the microwave.
- Gentle torso twists before you get in the car.
- A slow squat or two after you stand up from a chair.

These micro-movements add up. Over time, they reduce stiffness, improve circulation, and make your body feel more responsive.

Frictionless Movement Triggers

One of the biggest barriers to moving more is the hidden friction in your environment:

- The chair that's *just a little too comfortable.*
- The remote within easy reach.
- The habit of staying seated because everything you need is right there.

Frictionless triggers flip that script.
Examples:

- Keep a resistance band hanging near your desk as a visual cue.
- Place a small step or sturdy box where you walk past it often—so you can step up once or twice without thinking.
- Use reminders: set a timer to stand or stretch every 45 minutes.
- Store your most-used items in a higher cabinet to encourage reaching and squatting.

When movement becomes the easiest option, it becomes the

most likely.

Household Tasks as Hidden Training

You don't have to carve out extra hours to build strength and mobility.

Your home is already a gym, if you know how to see it:

- **Laundry baskets:** Carry them with good posture and core engagement.
- **Grocery bags:** Hold them evenly on both sides for balance.
- **Vacuuming or sweeping:** Use deliberate lunges to strengthen your legs.
- **Gardening:** Squat, hinge, reach, rotate—all the movements your body needs.

When you approach these everyday activities with intention, you transform chores into practice—and reclaim time that might otherwise slip away.

One Simple Commitment

If you take only one idea from this section, let it be this:

Movement doesn't have to be big to matter. It just has to be consistent.

Every posture reset, every mobility snack, every small choice to stand up or take a few steps is a vote for the kind of life you want to keep living.

In the next segment, we'll put this into a **simple four-week plan** to help you build momentum without overwhelm.

CHAPTER 6

Practice Plan: Weeks 1–4

By now, you understand why daily movement matters—and you've seen how small actions can have an outsized impact.

But even with the best intentions, new habits can feel overwhelming if you try to do everything at once.

That's why this plan is built to be **simple, flexible, and sustainable.**

You don't need perfection.

You just need to show up, one day at a time.

How This Practice Works

For the next four weeks, you'll focus on **three daily pillars:**

1. **Steps and Movement Minutes**
2. **Posture Awareness**
3. **Intentional Check-Ins**

These are the building blocks of Tier 1—your foundation of everyday vitality.

You can track them in a journal, on your phone, or with a wearable if you like. But you don't have to obsess. Progress is about trends over time, not hitting a number every single day.

Daily Steps and Movement Minutes
Why it matters:

Your body is designed to move frequently. Steps and gentle motion help lubricate joints, improve circulation, and keep your energy steady.

How to start:

- If you're mostly sedentary, aim for **3,000–4,000 steps per day** as your initial target.
- If you already walk regularly, set a goal to increase by **1,000–2,000 steps per day.**
- Remember: all movement counts—housework, errands, gentle strolls, dancing around the kitchen.

Posture Awareness
Why it matters:
Good posture isn't just about appearance. It affects breathing, circulation, and how your muscles engage. Frequent resets build muscle memory.
How to start:

- Choose **three anchor moments** in your day to reset your posture (for example: after waking, before lunch, before dinner).
- Each time, take **30 seconds** to:
- Lengthen your spine
- Soften your shoulders
- Breathe slowly

That's it. A few intentional breaths can transform how you feel.

Intentional Check-Ins
Why it matters:
You can't change what you don't notice. Daily check-ins bring awareness to your patterns.
How to start:
Once a day, pause and ask yourself:

- Have I been sitting too long?
- What could I do in the next few minutes to move more freely?
- How does my body feel right now?

Over time, this reflection becomes second nature—and you'll find yourself making micro-adjustments without even thinking.

A Simple Weekly Framework

Here's how you might structure your first four weeks:

Week 1:

- Focus on posture resets three times per day.
- Notice how often you sit for more than an hour without moving.

Week 2:

- Set your daily step target.
- Add one mobility snack (like ankle circles or shoulder rolls) each morning.

Week 3:

- Increase your movement minutes by 10–15% over Week 2.
- Start using a simple checklist to record your posture resets and step count.

Week 4:

- Choose one household task to turn into hidden training (like squatting while you fold laundry).
- Reflect on what has improved—energy, stiffness, mood.

Progress Over Perfection

Remember: This is not a contest. If you miss a day, nothing is lost.

Your body cares about what you do most of the time—not every once in a while.

Consistency is your real goal.

Gentleness is your best companion.

Next, we'll look at **what you'll start to notice as these habits take root.**

What You'll Notice

One of the quiet gifts of daily movement is that the benefits often arrive gently.

They don't always announce themselves with fireworks or dramatic changes. More often, they slip into your life in subtle ways—until one day, you realize you feel *different.*

More awake.

More capable.

More like yourself.

Here are some of the early signs you're on the right track:

A Steady Energy Boost

At first, you may feel a little tired as your body adapts to more movement. That's normal. Within a week or two, you'll likely notice your baseline energy starts to rise.

You might:

- Wake up feeling less stiff.
- Find it easier to get going in the morning.
- Feel steadier through the afternoon without the same crash.

Movement is like gently stoking a fire—each small action fuels your vitality.

Fewer Aches and Stiff Spots

When you stay in one position for long stretches, your body starts to feel like it's "settling in."

Daily movement interrupts that settling.

You may notice:

- Less tightness in your hips and shoulders.
- Fewer little pains when you stand up or turn.
- A sense of smoothness returning to your joints.

It doesn't take long for your body to remember that it *can* feel good.

Confidence in Everyday Tasks

Perhaps the most meaningful change is the return of quiet confidence:

- You get out of a chair without thinking.
- You carry bags without worrying about your back.
- You walk a little faster because it feels natural.

These ordinary moments are where fitness truly lives—not in the gym, but in the texture of your daily life.

A Subtle Shift in Identity

As these small wins accumulate, something even more important happens:

You start to see yourself differently.

You're no longer someone "trying to get moving."

You're someone who *moves*.

That shift in identity is powerful.

It makes consistency feel less like effort and more like an expression of who you are becoming.

What Happens Next

Tier 1—Daily Movement—lays the foundation.

It teaches your body to expect activity.

It creates the momentum you'll build on in the next layers of training.

So celebrate every bit of progress, no matter how small.

The first time you notice an ache is gone, or a task feels easier, pause and acknowledge it.

Because those are the moments that prove:

You're not stuck.

You're not past your prime.

You're in motion—and motion is life.

Chapter 7

Tier 2: Intentional Exercise – Strength and Resilience

The Sweet Spot of Training Intensity

Daily movement sets the stage.
It wakes up your body.
It restores basic mobility.
It reconnects you to a life that moves.

But if you want to build *more*—more strength, more resilience, more capacity to handle life's demands—you need something beyond everyday activity.

This is where **Intentional Exercise**—Tier 2—comes in.

Why Training Intensity Matters

At this stage of life, the question isn't whether you should train harder.

It's **how much is enough to spark growth—without tipping into fatigue or injury?**

Many people fall into two camps:

1. **The under-challenged:**

- Always keeping effort comfortable.
- Rarely testing strength or endurance.
- Staying stuck in the same place for years.

1. **The over-challenged:**

- Pushing too hard, too soon.
- Treating every workout like a test of willpower.
- Getting frustrated or injured, then stopping altogether.

The sweet spot lies right between those extremes.
Enough to grow—not enough to break.

Finding Your Personal Threshold

Your ideal training zone is unique. It depends on:

- Your current fitness baseline
- Your health history
- Your recovery capacity
- Your goals

A good rule of thumb:

- **Strength training:** Effort should feel like 6–8 out of 10. Challenging, but with good form.
- **Cardio training:** You can talk in short sentences but not sing. (This is often called *Zone 2*.)
- **Mobility work:** Comfortable range of motion, no pain.

If you finish a session feeling pleasantly worked, but not wiped out, you're probably right where you need to be.

The Role of Each Component
  Cardio:
Keeps your heart and lungs strong.

Improves endurance for everything you love—travel, hiking, long days on your feet.

Supports brain health and mood.
  Strength:
Preserves muscle mass, which declines naturally after 50.

Protects your bones and joints.

Builds confidence in your body's ability to handle real-world loads.
  Mobility:
Maintains healthy joints.

Reduces stiffness and injury risk.

Improves ease of movement in everyday life.

One Size Doesn't Fit All

Intentional Exercise isn't about copying someone else's routine.

It's about designing sessions that respect your life, your energy, and your purpose.

For some people, that might mean 3 short workouts each week.

For others, a mix of strength and brisk walking spread over more days.

What matters most is that you train **on purpose**, not by accident.

A Gentle Reminder

This isn't a race.

There is no finish line you have to cross by next month or next year.

There is only this question:

What can I do today that gently stretches my capacity—without overwhelming it?

If you can answer that, you've already found your sweet spot.

Your Weekly Framework

If Tier 1—daily movement—is the foundation, Tier 2 is where you begin to build something new.

Intentional Exercise isn't about doing the hardest thing you can imagine.

It's about choosing activities that safely challenge your body—*and fit into your real life.*

This section will give you a clear framework for the three pillars of structured training:

Zone 2 Cardio
Resistance Training
Mobility Flows

Let's walk through each piece so you know exactly what it looks like—and how to make it your own.

What is Zone 2 Cardio?

You'll hear trainers and articles throw around terms like *aerobic conditioning* or *steady-state cardio*.

All this really means is movement that:

- Elevates your heart rate moderately
- Lets you talk in short sentences, but not sing
- Can be sustained for at least 20–40 minutes

This is often called **Zone 2**, and it's one of the most powerful ways to build endurance, heart health, and metabolic fitness.

Examples of Zone 2 Cardio:

- Brisk walking (indoors, outdoors, or on a treadmill)
- Steady cycling (stationary or outdoor)
- Swimming at a comfortable pace
- Elliptical machine
- Rowing machine at moderate intensity
- Hiking on gentle terrain
- Low-impact dance classes
- Cross-country skiing
- Water aerobics

You don't have to pick just one—variety helps you stay engaged.

What is Resistance Training?

Resistance simply means **your muscles are working against some kind of load.**

That load could be:

- Your own bodyweight
- A resistance band
- Dumbbells or kettlebells
- Weight machines
- Cables or pulleys
- Sandbags or medicine balls

Examples of Resistance Exercises:

- **Bodyweight:** squats, lunges, wall push-ups, glute bridges, step-ups
- **Bands:** standing rows, lateral raises, chest presses, biceps curls
- **Dumbbells:** deadlifts, overhead presses, goblet squats
- **Machines:** leg press, lat pulldown, chest press

For many beginners, **bodyweight + resistance bands** is the simplest and safest place to start.

Resistance training doesn't have to feel intimidating. Think of it as teaching your muscles to stay awake and strong.

What is a Mobility Flow?

Mobility flows are structured sequences that take your joints through their healthy ranges of motion.

They:

- Improve flexibility
- Help prevent stiffness
- Teach better movement patterns
- Ease aches and pains

Examples of Mobility Movements:

- Cat-camel spine flexion/extension
- Hip circles and lunges
- Shoulder rolls and reaches
- Ankle and wrist circles
- Gentle yoga sequences

You don't need an hour-long routine—5–10 minutes a few times a week can work wonders.

Your Weekly Framework (Simple Version)

Here's a sustainable example schedule most people can adapt:

2–3 Cardio Sessions

- 20–40 minutes each
- Zone 2 intensity
- Walk, bike, swim, or any other steady movement you enjoy

2–3 Resistance Sessions

- 20–40 minutes each
- Focus on major muscle groups
- Alternate upper and lower body if you like

2–3 Mobility Sessions

- 5–15 minutes each
- Gentle, restorative

That's it—no complicated spreadsheets required.

What if You're Busy?

Here's an example **30-Minute Workout Structure** you can do at home or the gym:

1. **5 minutes:** Mobility warm-up (hip circles, shoulder rolls, gentle squats)
2. **10–15 minutes:** Resistance training circuit (e.g., squats,

rows, presses, planks)
3. **10–15 minutes:** Brisk cardio (treadmill walk, cycling, step-ups)
4. **Optional:** 3–5 minutes cool-down stretches

If you can only do 15–20 minutes, focus on the resistance part—strength is often the first capacity to fade, and it makes everything else easier.

How to Choose

You don't have to love every modality. But you should feel comfortable and safe.

Ask yourself:

- What am I most likely to stick with?
- What equipment do I have access to?
- What feels fun or satisfying?

You can—and should—experiment.

Remember: **the best plan is the one you'll actually do.**

Practice Plan: Weeks 5–8

You've built the foundation with daily movement.

You've learned what Intentional Exercise looks like.

Now, let's put it together into a **four-week plan** that guides you step by step.

Remember:

You don't have to be perfect. You don't have to follow this exactly.

These weeks are here to **give you structure**—not to box you in.

Adapt as needed.
Go at your pace.
Celebrate every small win.

How This Practice Works

For the next four weeks, you'll focus on three areas:

Cardio Targets
Resistance Basics
Joint Mobility Drills

The goal isn't to max out your capacity. The goal is to **establish consistency.**

Week 5: Foundations & Familiarity

Cardio:

- Choose 2 sessions of 20–30 minutes each.
- Keep it Zone 2 (moderate effort—you can talk but not sing).
- Examples: brisk walking, steady cycling, swimming.

Resistance:

- 2 short sessions this week.
- Focus on learning form and building confidence.
- Examples:
- Bodyweight squats (or sit-to-stand from a chair)
- Wall push-ups
- Resistance band rows

Mobility:

- 5–10 minutes daily.
- Simple movements: shoulder rolls, hip circles, gentle twisting.

Week 6: Adding Volume
Cardio:

- Increase to 3 sessions of 25–35 minutes.
- Try a new modality if you feel ready (e.g., elliptical or dance class).

Resistance:

- 2–3 sessions.
- Add one more exercise per session if you feel strong.
- Example: lunges, light dumbbell presses, band pull-aparts.

Mobility:

- Maintain daily practice.
- Spend extra time on any area that feels stiff.

Week 7: Building Confidence
Cardio:

- Maintain 3 sessions, or add an extra short walk on one additional day.
- Notice your recovery—are you less winded than when you started?

Resistance:

- 3 sessions if energy allows.
- Begin gently increasing resistance:
- More repetitions
- Slightly heavier weights or stronger bands

Mobility:

- Explore a simple flow sequence (like gentle yoga or tai chi-inspired moves).

Week 8: Reflect & Refine
Cardio:

- Keep 3 sessions.
- Try one longer session (40+ minutes) if you feel ready.

Resistance:

- 3 sessions.
- Focus on form quality and mindful movement.

Mobility:

- Use this week to notice which habits you enjoy—and which ones need adjustment.

A Few Reminders

- **Listen to your body.** Some soreness is normal, but sharp pain is not.
- **Rest is part of the plan.** Take 1–2 full rest days per week.
- **Consistency beats intensity.** Showing up regularly matters more than pushing hard.

Reflection Questions

At the end of Week 8, pause and ask yourself:

- What has changed in how I feel?
- Which exercises felt best?
- What do I want to build on next month?

Your answers will help you shape your next steps with clarity and confidence.

Wins to Look For

Sometimes, progress in fitness can feel invisible—especially when you're focused on the scale or arbitrary numbers.

But the truth is, real wins show up in **how you feel** and **what you can do.**

When you train consistently, you'll start to notice subtle shifts that build your confidence and prove you're moving in the right direction.

Here are a few signs to celebrate:

A Stronger Heart and Lungs (VO_2 Max)

VO_2 max is a fancy term for how well your body uses oxygen during exercise.

When it improves, you might notice:

- You recover faster after walking up stairs.
- You can carry groceries without feeling out of breath.
- Your heart rate comes back down more quickly after activity.

Even modest improvements here are strongly linked to better health and longer life.

Remember: You don't have to hit elite levels—*any* upward trend is meaningful.

Steadier Balance

Balance is easy to take for granted—until you start to lose it.

As you practice resistance and mobility exercises, you may notice:

- You can stand on one leg a little longer.
- You feel more stable stepping off curbs or reaching overhead.
- You recover from a trip or stumble without panic.

These are huge wins. They mean your nervous system and muscles are working together more effectively.

More Strength (and Confidence)

Strength doesn't always announce itself dramatically. Sometimes it shows up like this:

- You get up off the floor without using your hands.
- You move a heavy object and realize it felt easier.

- You notice muscle definition in places you hadn't before.

These moments matter.

They remind you that your body is still adaptable. Still capable. Still ready for more.

More Energy, Less Aches

Many people start to feel:

- Less morning stiffness
- Fewer little pains when they move
- A steady, satisfying energy that lasts all day

This is your body thanking you for showing up.

A Quiet Sense of Pride

Perhaps the most important win of all is the shift you feel inside:

- You start to see yourself as someone who trains.
- You trust your body a little more each week.
- You notice your mindset changing from "Can I do this?" to "What else can I do?"

Celebrate every sign of progress—no matter how small it seems.

These are the milestones that prove your effort is working.
You're building not just strength, but resilience.
Not just fitness, but freedom.

Chapter 8

Tier 3: Performance Training (Power, Precision, and Flow)

What High-Level Function Looks Like at 60+

When you hear the words **"high-level function,"** you might picture elite athletes or lifelong performers—people who have always been training, who somehow stayed perfectly fit.

But here's the truth:

High-level function is not reserved for the genetically blessed or the endlessly disciplined.

It's available to you—in your own way, on your own timeline—if you build toward it with consistency and care.

What Does High-Level Function Mean?

By the time most people reach their 60s or 70s, the expectations are often depressingly low:

- Get up and down without help.

- Take slow, careful steps.
- Avoid falling.

That is not your ceiling.

High-level function at any age means:

Agility – the ability to change direction quickly and safely.

Power – the capacity to produce force when you need it (like catching yourself if you trip).

Coordination – smooth, efficient movement across multiple joints and muscle groups.

Focus – the mental clarity to respond rather than react.

When you combine these qualities, you get a life that feels dynamic, capable, and fully yours.

Agility: Moving with Ease and Quickness

Agility isn't about sprinting across a soccer field—unless you want it to be.

It's about:

- Navigating uneven sidewalks without hesitation.
- Shifting your weight confidently when you step sideways.
- Turning, reaching, or pivoting with balance.

As you train, agility shows up in ordinary moments. You'll notice you don't have to "think" about every step—you simply move.

Power: Strength in Motion

Power is strength applied quickly.

It's the difference between *slowly* standing up and *springing* to your feet.

Why does this matter? Because real life often requires speed:

- Catching yourself mid-fall.
- Lifting a heavy object before it slips.
- Climbing stairs without slowing down.

Power is one of the first capacities to decline as we age—and one of the most important to reclaim. Even small improvements in lower-body power can dramatically reduce fall risk and improve confidence.

Coordination: Moving Smoothly and Efficiently

Coordination is what lets you:

- Carry a load without wobbling.
- Perform complex tasks like gardening, dancing, or playing with grandkids.
- Feel graceful instead of clumsy.

When you train for coordination, you teach your nervous system to sequence muscles in the right order, at the right time.

This is part of why balance drills, mobility flows, and integrated strength exercises are so valuable: they rebuild the patterns that let you move as a unified whole.

Focus: The Mental Edge

High-level function isn't just physical.

It's the **mental presence** that allows you to respond skillfully in the moment.

- Noticing the obstacle in your path before you trip over it.

- Staying calm if you lose your balance.
- Feeling fully engaged in your body instead of distracted or tense.

This kind of focus isn't reserved for martial artists or elite performers.

It's trainable.

It begins with simple awareness—choosing to be *present* when you move.

What's Possible?

If you've never trained for agility, power, coordination, and focus, it can feel almost impossible to imagine yourself moving that way.

But I promise you this:

You are capable of far more than you think.

I've seen people in their 60s, 70s, and beyond:

- Master kettlebell swings and gentle plyometrics.
- Learn tai chi forms that improve balance and fluidity.
- Build enough power to climb hills with ease.
- Develop the confidence to hike, travel, and play again.

They didn't get there overnight. They started exactly where you are now—by believing improvement was possible.

And then they took one step, and another, and another.

A Vision for Your Next Chapter

So before you worry about sets, reps, or techniques, take a moment to simply imagine this:

You move with ease.

You feel quick on your feet.

You trust your body to support you in any environment.

You feel strong, capable, and quietly proud.

This is what high-level function can look like in your 60s and beyond.

And it's not a fantasy.

It's the natural outcome of showing up for yourself, again and again, with patience and purpose.

Advanced Movement Integration

If Tier 1 was about waking up your body...

...and Tier 2 was about building strength and endurance...

Tier 3 is about weaving everything together.

This is where your training becomes more than the sum of its parts—where strength, balance, breath, and focus combine into something that feels powerful and natural.

Why Integration Matters

Most traditional exercise programs isolate qualities:

- Strength training here.
- Cardio there.
- Balance and mobility somewhere else.

But in real life, everything happens *at once.*

You rarely get to say:

"Hold on, let me only use my quads for this next movement."

You have to lift, stabilize, breathe, and think—often under mild pressure or unexpected circumstances.

Advanced Movement Integration prepares you for exactly that.

It's what turns raw strength into usable capability.

Combining Strength, Balance, and Breath

Here's the heart of integrated training:

Strength gives you the power to move with purpose.

Balance helps you control and direct that power.

Breath keeps your nervous system calm and steady.

When you train these elements together, you build *real-world readiness.*

Examples of Integrated Exercises:

- **Loaded Carries:** Holding a weight in one hand while you walk. Strengthens grip, builds core stability, trains posture.
- **Split Squats or Lunges:** Combines lower-body strength, balance, and coordination. Teaches you to control movement through space.
- **Kettlebell Swings:** Trains power, timing, and breath control.
- **Turkish Get-Ups:** A full-body challenge requiring strength, balance, and focus.
- **Single-Leg Deadlifts:** Builds posterior chain strength and intense stability.

You don't need to master every movement. You just need to practice combining qualities in ways that feel safe and appropriately challenging.

Breathing as a Performance Tool

By this point in the book, you already know that breath shapes how you feel and how you move.

In integrated training, breath is the bridge between tension and control:

- **Inhale** to gather stability before lifting or lowering.
- **Exhale** to create bracing and focus during exertion.
- **Calm breathing** between sets to reset your nervous system.

This isn't fancy or esoteric. It's practical. The more comfortable you get with intentional breathing, the more power and steadiness you'll feel.

Training Under Mild Stress (The Power of Stakes)

There's another element to integration that matters deeply: **training with a sense of stakes.**

You don't need to simulate an emergency. But you do need *just enough challenge* to keep you engaged and alert.

Here are a few ways to do it safely:

- **Timed sets:** Instead of counting reps, work for 30–45 seconds, maintaining good form under a little time pressure.
- **Unstable surfaces:** Perform balance exercises on a foam pad or soft mat to create natural variability.
- **Cognitive dual-tasking:** Count backward by threes while you hold a plank. Recite a grocery list while you balance on one leg.
- **Mini-obstacles:** Step over low barriers while carrying light weights to mimic real-world demands.

This isn't about making things harder for the sake of it.

It's about practicing your skills in slightly unpredictable

conditions—so you're more prepared when life throws you a curveball.

Real-World Carryover
This approach has a powerful ripple effect:

- You'll feel more comfortable navigating uneven ground.
- You'll recover balance faster if you trip.
- You'll stay calmer under pressure.

It's not about becoming perfect.
It's about creating a body—and a mindset—that can adapt.

Advanced Movement Integration is where training stops feeling like isolated exercises—and starts feeling like life.

Practice Plan: Weeks 9-12

By now, you've built a strong foundation:
Daily movement (Tier 1)
Intentional exercise (Tier 2)
A growing confidence in what your body can do
In this final phase, you'll begin weaving everything together: power, balance, mobility, and focus.

Important:
This is not about pushing yourself to exhaustion.
This is about exploring your capacity—gently and consistently.
You don't need to do everything perfectly.
You just need to keep showing up with curiosity and care.

How This Practice Works

Over the next four weeks, you'll introduce:

Plyometrics: Simple, low-impact power exercises

Reaction Drills: Quick-response movements to sharpen coordination

Integrated Mobility + Load: Complex exercises that challenge multiple systems at once

You can layer these into your usual weekly framework or dedicate one session per week to advanced practice.

If you have any health concerns, check with your doctor or physical therapist before starting this phase.

Week 9: Introducing Power and Reaction

Plyometrics:

- **Mini Squat Hops:**
- Start with a quarter squat.
- Hop gently, landing softly.
- 2–3 sets of 6–10 reps.
- **Alternatives:**
- Step-ups performed quickly but under control.

Reaction Drills:

- **Toss and Catch:**
- Toss a tennis ball against a wall and catch it.
- Try catching with one hand.
- **Alternatives:**
- Have a partner call out directions while you step or pivot.

Integrated Mobility + Load:

- **Suitcase Carries:**
- Hold a weight in one hand, walk 20–30 feet.
- Keep your torso upright and steady.

Week 10: Building Complexity
Plyometrics:

- **Gentle Lateral Hops:**
- Hop side to side over a line or cone.
- Focus on balance and soft landings.

Reaction Drills:

- **Quick Step Taps:**
- Place a small object on the floor.
- Step to tap it lightly and return to start as quickly as possible.

Integrated Mobility + Load:

- **Lunge with Rotation:**
- Lunge forward, rotate your torso gently toward the front knee.
- Return to standing.

Week 11: Combining Elements
Plyometrics:

- **Box Step-Offs:**
- Step off a low platform or step, landing softly.

- Focus on balance and control.

Reaction Drills:

- **Pattern Recall:**
- Tap four points on the floor in a memorized sequence.
- Repeat, adding speed.

Integrated Mobility + Load:

- **Single-Leg Deadlift:**
- Hold light weight, hinge forward on one leg.
- Return to standing with control.

Week 12: Reflection and Progress
Plyometrics:

- Choose your favorite exercise and repeat with improved form.

Reaction Drills:

- Combine footwork and catching (e.g., step-tap while tossing a ball).

Integrated Mobility + Load:

- Practice a mini "flow":
- Lunge with rotation → Suitcase Carry → Single-Leg Balance

Tips for Success
Start small. Even a few reps build skill.
Focus on form over speed. Quality always wins.
Rest when needed. Recovery is still part of the work.
Celebrate every improvement.

A Gentle Reminder
If you feel intimidated by these exercises, remember:
You've already built the foundation.

You have the strength, balance, and awareness to explore more dynamic movement.

Every step you take here is about proving to yourself that growth is still possible.

Mental-Physical Synergy

By now, you've probably noticed that training isn't only about your muscles, heart, or joints.

It's also about your **mind.**

This is the hidden dimension that transforms exercise from a chore into a practice—something that nourishes not just your body, but your sense of meaning and self-respect.

When you bring your full attention into your training, you create something powerful:

Mental-Physical Synergy.

The Power of Cognitive Focus
Every rep you do has two parts:

- The movement itself

- The *awareness* you bring to it

Research shows that when you pay attention to how your body feels and what it's doing, you:
Recruit more muscle fibers
Strengthen neuromuscular connections
Improve learning and retention
Reduce injury risk
This is called **purposeful repetition.**
It means you're not just counting reps—you're *inhabiting* them.

What Does Purposeful Repetition Look Like?

Here are simple ways to apply it:

- Feel the tension in the working muscle.
- Notice where you're bracing or compensating.
- Breathe deliberately as you move.
- Move with the intention to learn, not just to finish.

A set of 10 mindless squats is simply time spent.
A set of 5 focused squats is practice that changes you.

Martial Presence

In martial arts, there is a principle called **zanshin**—a state of relaxed, total awareness.
It's not hypervigilance.
It's not zoning out.
It's the feeling of being fully present, eyes open, mind clear.
You can cultivate this in any practice:

- In a balance drill, feel the micro-adjustments of your feet.
- In a carry or lunge, sense your center of gravity moving through space.
- In a reaction drill, notice the split-second decisions your body makes.

This presence builds confidence.

It teaches you to trust yourself under mild stress.

It creates the foundation for what athletes call *flow.*

Flow State: Your Body and Mind as One

Flow is that rare, beautiful experience when:

- Your skills meet the challenge perfectly
- You lose track of time
- You feel fully immersed in the task

While flow can't be forced, you can create the conditions for it:

Choose tasks that are challenging but within your reach

Remove distractions (phones, background noise)

Set a clear goal for the session

Pay attention to each moment

Flow doesn't just feel good—it's also where your biggest gains often happen.

Peak Performance Principles

You don't have to be an elite athlete to benefit from the same principles they use:

1. **Clarity:** Know why you're here today. Even a simple goal—*move with good form, breathe calmly*—is enough.

2. **Presence:** Keep your mind where your body is.
3. **Feedback:** Notice how things feel. Adjust without judgment.
4. **Challenge:** Stretch your capacity a little bit, but not to the breaking point.

A New Relationship to Training

When you approach your sessions this way, exercise stops being something you *have* to do.

It becomes:

- A moving meditation
- A rehearsal for real life
- A celebration of your capacity

And it reinforces a deeper truth:

Your mind and body are not separate.

They are partners in the project of becoming stronger, steadier, and more fully alive.

Your Physical Legacy

If you've read this far, you've already proven something important about yourself:

You are not willing to let your life shrink.

You understand that fitness isn't about chasing youth or impressing anyone else.

It's about **protecting your freedom.**

It's about **honoring your potential.**

And it's about building something you can carry forward into every year ahead.

More Than Ability

Most people think of training only in terms of *capacity*:

- How strong am I?
- How fast am I?
- How flexible am I?

Those things matter. But they're only part of the story.

The real gift of consistent movement is the way it shapes your **identity.**

With every session, you're telling yourself:

- *I am someone who shows up.*
- *I am someone who learns.*
- *I am someone who doesn't give up.*

This identity is the foundation for confidence.

Because when you prove to yourself—again and again—that you can keep going, you stop questioning whether you're capable.

You start *trusting* that you are.

The Confidence to Engage

Fitness isn't measured by what you can lift or how far you can run.

It's measured by how willing you feel to engage with life.

- To travel, knowing you can handle the stairs and the lug-

gage.
- To garden or play with your grandkids, knowing you won't be too sore to enjoy it.
- To get down on the floor—and back up again—without hesitation.

These moments are your real legacy.

They are proof that you didn't let fear or inertia define what was possible for you.

A Capacity That Grows With You

One of the greatest misconceptions about aging is that decline is inevitable and irreversible.

Yes, change is inevitable.

But decline is not the only option.

The choices you make now—about how you move, how you recover, and how you think—create a momentum that carries forward.

Your capacity doesn't disappear the moment you turn 70 or 80.

It adapts.

It evolves.

It reflects the habits you've practiced over decades.

What You Leave Behind

Your physical legacy isn't just about you.

It's also about the example you set for the people you love:

- Showing that growth is possible at any age.
- Modeling resilience and self-respect.
- Proving that it's never too late to care for yourself.

When your kids, grandkids, friends, and community see you moving with purpose, they see what's possible for them, too.

That's a powerful gift.

A Closing Thought

If you take only one message from this chapter, let it be this: **Your body is worth the effort.**

Not because you're trying to avoid getting older.

But because you're choosing to live fully, with whatever time you have.

That choice—over and over again—is how you build a legacy of strength, confidence, and freedom.

Chapter 9

Nutrition and Supplementation for Longevity & Performance

Nutrition for Training and Recovery

Let's start with a simple truth that cuts through all the noise:

You can't out-train a bad diet.

No matter how dedicated you are to movement, if your body isn't getting the nutrients it needs, you'll eventually feel it—lower energy, slower recovery, stalled progress, and sometimes even injury.

But here's something equally important to remember:

There is no perfect diet that works for everyone.

If you've ever felt confused because respected experts disagree, you're not alone. Some advocate high-fat, low-carb. Others insist on plant-based eating. Still others emphasize ancient eating patterns or modern meal timing strategies.

The truth is simpler—and more hopeful—than it seems.

Human beings are remarkably adaptable. Throughout history,

people have thrived on widely varied diets. From the plant-heavy traditions of Okinawa to the hearty, animal-rich diets of the Arctic, what matters most isn't a label. It's **how you nourish yourself consistently.**

Why Diet Matters More As You Age

In your 20s and 30s, you can get away with a lot—missed meals, low-quality food, inconsistent eating patterns. But after 50, your body's resilience starts to change.

Protein synthesis slows.

Recovery takes longer.

Blood sugar and insulin sensitivity become more sensitive to what you eat.

Digestive processes shift.

In other words, food becomes more than fuel. It's part of your **daily recovery strategy.**

Nutrition is what rebuilds your muscles after training, balances hormones, supports your immune system, and provides the raw materials for energy and focus.

The Synergy Between Food and Training

One of the most powerful things you can do for yourself is see nutrition and movement as partners.

When you move with intention, your body sends a signal: **Repair. Rebuild. Grow.**

When you nourish yourself well, you provide the building blocks to answer that call.

Think of it this way:

- **Training creates demand.**
- **Food meets that demand.**

- **Recovery completes the cycle.**

This synergy is especially crucial if you're working to maintain muscle mass, improve cardiovascular capacity, or sustain mobility. Without adequate nutrition, your training simply can't deliver its full benefits.

Gut Health, Protein Synthesis, and Energy Availability

Three areas deserve special attention as you age:

Gut Health

Your digestive system affects everything—nutrient absorption, inflammation, immunity, even mood. A diet rich in fiber, varied plant foods, and fermented options (like sauerkraut, kimchi, or yogurt if you tolerate dairy) can help keep your microbiome diverse and robust.

Protein Synthesis

Muscle doesn't just maintain itself. After 50, your body becomes less efficient at using dietary protein to repair and grow muscle tissue. Research shows that spreading protein intake evenly across meals can help—think 20–30 grams per meal rather than one large serving at dinner.

Energy Availability

If you're consistently under-eating, whether because of appetite changes, busyness, or intentional restriction, your energy will suffer. Your body needs carbohydrates, fats, and protein to power training and recovery.

This isn't about eating "perfectly." It's about eating **sufficiently**—enough to support your goals and feel steady.

A Respectful Invitation

Here's what I want you to take away from this chapter:

You don't have to choose one dogma.
You don't have to label yourself.
You don't have to get it exactly right every day.

You simply need to be curious, pay attention to what nourishes you, and respect the role food plays in your training and recovery.

Because the choices you make in the kitchen are every bit as important as the ones you make in the gym or on the mat.

No One-Size-Fits-All: Adapting to Your Diet Philosophy

One of the biggest barriers people face when trying to improve their nutrition is the feeling that they have to pick a side.

You've probably noticed it yourself:

- Entire books and podcasts insisting that *this* way of eating is the only right way.
- Friends or relatives swearing by one approach and dismissing all the others.
- Social media amplifying every disagreement into an all-or-nothing war of ideas.

Here's what I believe:

Most dietary philosophies can work if you approach them with respect, curiosity, and consistency.

Some people thrive on a plant-based diet. Others feel their best with higher fat intake. Some find clarity in tracking macros, while others prefer intuitive eating.

This is your body. Your life. Your choice.

The only requirement is that your diet supports:

Enough energy to fuel your movement

Sufficient protein to protect your muscle

The nutrients your body needs to recover, repair, and stay vital

Let's look at a few common approaches, without judgment or hype, so you can see which feels most aligned with your goals and values.

Keto & Low-Carb Approaches

What it is:

A diet that severely restricts carbohydrates, emphasizing fats as the primary fuel source.

Potential Benefits:

- More stable blood sugar for some people
- Reduced hunger due to higher fat intake
- Can help some lose weight and improve metabolic markers

Considerations:

- May be harder to get sufficient fiber and certain micronutrients
- Some experience fatigue or reduced performance in high-intensity training
- Needs careful planning to avoid excessive saturated fat

Tips for Active Adults Over 50:

- Prioritize healthy fats (olive oil, avocado, nuts) over processed sources
- Ensure adequate non-starchy vegetables for fiber and an-

tioxidants
- Watch protein intake—too little can accelerate muscle loss

Mediterranean Diet
What it is:

A flexible, plant-forward diet emphasizing whole grains, legumes, vegetables, fruit, fish, and olive oil.

Potential Benefits:

- Strong research backing for cardiovascular health and longevity
- High in fiber and healthy fats
- Sustainable for most lifestyles

Considerations:

- Some find the moderate carbohydrate intake less compatible with strict low-carb goals
- May require planning if you don't enjoy seafood

Tips for Active Adults Over 50:

- Aim for protein at each meal (fish, legumes, eggs)
- Focus on variety—different colors, textures, and nutrient sources
- Use extra virgin olive oil liberally as your main fat

Vegan & Vegetarian Diets
What it is:

Eating patterns that exclude (vegan) or limit (vegetarian) animal products.

Potential Benefits:

- High in fiber, vitamins, and antioxidants
- Can reduce inflammation markers
- Often easier to maintain a healthy weight

Considerations:

- Needs careful planning to get enough protein, vitamin B12, iron, and omega-3s
- May require supplementation

Tips for Active Adults Over 50:

- Prioritize legumes, tofu, tempeh, and high-protein grains
- Consider B12, vitamin D, and algae-based omega-3 supplements
- Keep an eye on total calorie intake if appetite is low

Paleo & Ancestral Diets
What it is:
A diet modeled after pre-agricultural eating—meats, fish, vegetables, fruits, nuts, seeds—excluding grains, legumes, and most dairy.

Potential Benefits:

- High in protein and micronutrients
- Less processed food

- Often naturally lower in sugar

Considerations:

- Can be expensive and restrictive for some
- Excluding grains and legumes may reduce beneficial fiber if not replaced with other sources

Tips for Active Adults Over 50:

- Emphasize a wide variety of vegetables and tubers for carbs and fiber
- Choose lean meats and fatty fish over processed meats
- Ensure sufficient calcium (dark greens, almonds, mineral-rich water)

Other Approaches (Intermittent Fasting, Intuitive Eating, Flexitarian)
What it is:

- **Intermittent Fasting:** Cycling periods of eating and fasting
- **Intuitive Eating:** Listening to hunger/fullness cues without strict rules
- **Flexitarian:** Mostly plant-based with occasional animal products

Potential Benefits:

- Greater flexibility
- Encourages mindfulness and body awareness

- Can fit many lifestyles

Considerations:

- Fasting windows may be tricky if you train early in the day
- Some need more structure to maintain protein and calorie intake

Tips for Active Adults Over 50:

- Ensure you're meeting energy and protein needs within your eating windows
- Use a food journal to spot patterns if intuitive eating feels vague
- Give yourself permission to adjust as your needs change

How to Choose

Rather than picking a "perfect" diet, ask yourself:

1. **Does this approach support my training and recovery?**
2. **Does it feel sustainable and nourishing?**
3. **Am I getting enough protein, fiber, healthy fats, and micronutrients?**
4. **Does it align with my values and preferences?**

A Respectful Invitation

Remember:

You don't need to convince anyone else your way is best.

And you don't have to defend your choices to anyone, including yourself.

The only test that matters is:

Is this working for me?

9.3 – Supplementation as Support

If you spend any time in health and fitness circles, you'll quickly see a familiar promise:

"This supplement is the missing piece."

While some products can genuinely help, it's important to remember:

Supplements are just that—supplements.

They are not a substitute for real food, consistent movement, or quality sleep.

But used thoughtfully, they can fill gaps, speed recovery, and help you stay strong and resilient as you age.

Common Nutrient Gaps Over 50

After 50, your body becomes less efficient at absorbing and using certain nutrients. Even if you eat well, some shortfalls are surprisingly common:

Vitamin D

Your skin's ability to synthesize vitamin D from sunlight decreases. This vitamin is critical for bone health, immune function, and mood.

Calcium

Bone density naturally declines, and many people—especially those avoiding dairy—fall short on calcium intake.

Vitamin B12

Absorption of B12, essential for nerve function and energy, decreases due to changes in stomach acid production.

Magnesium

Important for muscle relaxation, sleep quality, and cardiovascular health.

Protein

Not technically a "nutrient gap," but inadequate protein intake is common and contributes to muscle loss.

Role of Key Supplements

Below is a non-exhaustive look at some supplements worth discussing with your healthcare provider. Remember: not everyone needs everything, and more is not always better.

Creatine

Why it matters:

- Helps preserve muscle mass and strength, even in older adults.
- Supports short bursts of power and may benefit cognition.*Typical dose:*
- 3–5 grams daily.*Consider:*
- Generally safe for healthy kidneys, but always check with your doctor if you have kidney issues.

Omega-3 Fatty Acids (Fish Oil or Algae Oil)

Why it matters:

- Supports cardiovascular health, reduces inflammation, and may aid joint comfort.

Typical dose:

- 1–2 grams EPA + DHA combined daily.

Consider:

- Look for third-party tested products to avoid contaminants.

Vitamin D

Why it matters:

- Vital for bone density and immune health.

Typical dose:

- Varies widely—commonly 1,000–2,000 IU per day, but best determined by blood test.

Consider:

- Too much can be harmful—test levels periodically.

Magnesium

Why it matters:

- Supports muscle recovery, relaxation, and sleep.

Typical dose:

- 200–400 mg daily, preferably magnesium glycinate or citrate.

Consider:

- High doses may cause digestive upset.

Electrolytes

Why it matters:

- Replaces sodium, potassium, and magnesium lost in sweat, especially if training in heat.

How to use:

- Occasional electrolyte drinks or tablets can help maintain hydration.

Protein Supplements (Whey, Pea, Rice, etc.)

Why it matters:

- Convenient way to increase total protein intake.

How to use:

- 20–30 grams per serving as needed.

Consider:

- Look for minimal-ingredient options without excessive added sugars.

Finding Out What You Need

Before you stock up on bottles, pause and assess.

How do you know what you really need?

Bloodwork

Ask your doctor for labs that check:

- Vitamin D levels
- B12 status
- Iron, if fatigue is an issue
- Lipid and glucose markers

Consultation

A registered dietitian or a physician familiar with sports nutrition can help interpret results and design a plan.

Trial and Error

Sometimes, the only way to know if a supplement helps is to try it consistently for a few weeks and observe how you feel.

A Word of Caution

Not all supplements are created equal.

- Look for products verified by third-party testing organizations (e.g., NSF Certified for Sport, Informed Choice, USP Verified).
- Be wary of anything promising dramatic results.
- Remember that "natural" doesn't always mean safe.

A Respectful Perspective

You don't need to turn your kitchen counter into a pharmacy to age well.

But thoughtful supplementation—rooted in real evidence, guided by your unique needs—can be an elegant way to support your training, recovery, and daily vitality.

9.4 - Alcohol, Hormones, and Special Considerations

Nutrition isn't only about what you eat.

It's also about how you live—and how the choices you make outside the kitchen impact your training, recovery, and long-term health.

This section isn't here to tell you what you *must* do. It's here to give you information—so you can make choices with your eyes open and your values clear.

The Effects of Alcohol

For many, alcohol is woven into daily life—social connection, relaxation, ritual.

But it's worth knowing how it interacts with your goals:

Training and Recovery:

- Alcohol can impair muscle protein synthesis for up to 24–48 hours after a workout.
- It may blunt gains in strength and endurance, especially when consumed in larger amounts.

Sleep Quality:

- While alcohol can make you drowsy, it disrupts restorative deep sleep and increases nighttime awakenings.
- Over time, this impacts recovery, mood, and energy.

Metabolism and Body Composition:

- Alcohol is calorie-dense (7 calories per gram) and easily stored as fat.
- It can disrupt blood sugar balance and increase cravings.

A Balanced Perspective:

You don't have to quit entirely if you enjoy alcohol, but consider:

- Limiting intake around heavy training days
- Aiming for moderation (1 drink or fewer per day)
- Choosing alcohol-free days to support recovery

Introduction to Hormone Therapy

After 50, hormone levels naturally decline. For some people, this contributes to:

- Fatigue
- Reduced muscle mass
- Mood changes
- Lower libido

Hormone Replacement Therapy (HRT) can be helpful for select individuals—but it is not a panacea and carries risks.

Key Points to Know:
What It Is:

- In men, primarily testosterone replacement.
- In women, estrogen and/or progesterone therapy, espe-

cially around menopause.

Who It's For:

- People with clinically low hormone levels confirmed by blood tests.
- Those experiencing significant symptoms impacting daily life.

Cautions:

- Potential risks include cardiovascular issues, prostate or breast health concerns, and clotting disorders.
- Should always be supervised by a qualified physician with experience prescribing and monitoring hormone therapy.

If you're curious:
Ask your healthcare provider for comprehensive testing and discuss the full range of options.

Anti-Aging Fads vs. Tested Strategies

In recent years, a whole industry has emerged promising to "hack" aging with pills, injections, and miracle protocols.

Some claims are grounded in real science.

Others are…less so.

Red Flags to Watch For:

Big promises with no evidence

Expensive subscription programs that feel like pressure sales

Claims that one product will "reverse aging"

Strategies that *do* have strong evidence:

Regular resistance and aerobic exercise

Sufficient protein and micronutrients
Consistent, high-quality sleep
Stress management
Meaningful social connection
No supplement or therapy can replace these foundations.

A Thoughtful Approach
Aging is not a problem to solve.
It's a natural process to respect—and support as best you can.
Your job isn't to chase youth.
It's to build a body and lifestyle that serve you *now*.

Summary
Before we close, let's tie this chapter together:

- **Nutrition is foundational.** You can't out-train poor fuel.
- **No one diet is right for everyone.** Your best approach is the one you can sustain.
- **Supplements can help—but they are support, not salvation.**
- **Alcohol, hormones, and anti-aging protocols deserve thoughtful consideration.**

Most importantly:
You are allowed to choose what aligns with your goals, values, and lived experience.
The best strategy is the one you'll actually enjoy and practice consistently.

Chapter 10

Movement Based Arts and Practices

Movement Arts as a Lifelong Path

By now, you've seen that movement is more than a strategy to stay fit.

It's a way to reclaim your energy, protect your independence, and remember who you are.

But some forms of movement go even further.

They offer a framework for living.

Yoga, dance, and martial arts are not just workouts.

They are practices—living traditions that have helped people of every age stay strong, capable, and connected to something larger than themselves.

Unlike many modern sports, which are often centered on competition and youth, these movement arts were designed—or evolved—to be practiced across the lifespan.

In them, you'll find a rare combination:

Strength and power

Flexibility and grace

Mental focus and clarity

A community of people who understand that mastery is measured in decades, not weeks

Accessible and Valuable at Any Age

What makes these disciplines so unique is that they *welcome* you at any stage of life.

You don't have to be young.

You don't have to be especially fit or talented.

You don't have to have years of experience.

You simply have to be willing to begin.

Yoga can meet you on the mat whether you're 25 or 85.

Dance can be slow and meditative or vibrant and dynamic.

Martial arts can start as simple patterns of movement and grow into a lifelong study.

In each case, the practice adapts to you—not the other way around.

Strength, Flexibility, Coordination, and Inner Balance

These traditions are often described as "holistic," and for good reason:

- **Strength** is built through repeated, mindful effort—holding a yoga posture, practicing a dance phrase, or drilling a martial technique.
- **Flexibility** comes not only in your muscles and joints, but in your willingness to stay open to learning.
- **Coordination** is refined over years, through patterns that become second nature.
- **Inner balance** emerges as you learn to match breath with motion, intention with action.

Few other activities blend these elements so seamlessly.

Respecting the Elder Practitioner

One of the most beautiful aspects of movement arts is their reverence for experience.

In many martial arts, older practitioners are not seen as "past their prime." They are honored as living archives of skill, discipline, and wisdom.

The same is true in yoga communities and dance traditions around the world:

- Elders are recognized for their depth, not just their physical abilities.
- Their example shows that growth doesn't stop because the body ages—it simply shifts.

If you've ever worried that you're "too old to start," I invite you to look at these traditions differently:

They expect you to continue.

They *welcome* you to begin—right where you are, with the body you have today.

A Different Way to Measure Progress

So much of modern fitness is measured in numbers:

- Pounds lifted
- Miles run
- Calories burned

Movement arts offer a different metric:

How do you feel in your body?

How well can you direct your attention?
How gracefully can you respond to challenge?
These are the questions that guide you deeper, year after year.

A Quiet Invitation

If you've been looking for something more than exercise—something that feeds your mind and spirit as well as your body—consider exploring one of these traditions.

You don't have to become a master.

You don't have to commit for life.

You just have to be open to discovering what's possible when movement becomes a practice instead of a task.

Adapting the Practice to Your Season of Life

One of the reasons movement arts have endured across centuries is that they were never designed to be static.

They were built to grow with you.

When you're young, you may be drawn to speed, challenge, and ambition.

When you're older, the same practice naturally becomes slower, deeper, and more mindful.

This evolution isn't a loss.

It's a profound transformation—one that many lifelong practitioners come to cherish even more than their early years of training.

How Practice Evolves Over Time

In the beginning, you may focus on learning shapes:

- How to align your body in a yoga pose
- Where to step in a dance sequence
- How to coordinate breath and movement in a kata or form

But as the years pass, your attention shifts:

- The external shape becomes less important than the *quality* of your attention.
- The pace softens, but your awareness sharpens.
- The purpose moves from performance to presence.

In this way, movement arts are perfectly suited for midlife and beyond.

They invite you to practice in a way that respects your body's current capacity while still expanding what is possible.

Gentle Doesn't Mean Weak

Many people assume that "gentler" training means you're giving up on progress.

But in these traditions, gentle does not mean fragile.

It means:

- Moving with intention rather than compulsion.
- Honoring your limitations without surrendering to them.
- Finding strength in calm, steady effort.

You may no longer explode into jumps or drop into deep lunges—but you can refine your technique, improve your control, and develop an internal power that doesn't fade with age.

In fact, many elder practitioners describe this stage as their most rewarding. They've discovered that true mastery is not about force—it's about economy, subtlety, and grace.

Staying Active Without Burnout

When you train in your 20s or 30s, intensity is often the default.

But after 50, sustainability becomes the priority.

You start to ask different questions:

- How does this practice support my life outside the studio?
- Am I recovering fully between sessions?
- Is this adding to my well-being or draining it?

The art becomes one of consistency over intensity.

Show up often, not perfectly.

Keep your practice alive, even if it looks simpler.

That steadiness is what allows you to stay engaged for decades, rather than burning out or getting hurt.

A Practice That Meets You Where You Are

Whether you're stepping onto a yoga mat, a dance floor, or a martial arts dojo, remember:

You don't have to keep up with anyone else.

You don't have to measure your worth by the depth of a squat or the height of a kick.

You only have to ask:

- What does my body need today?
- What is my mind ready to explore?
- What would it feel like to practice with curiosity instead of judgment?

In this season of life, your practice is no longer about proving something.

It's about nourishing yourself.

Honoring your experience.

And finding joy in simply moving.

Physical, Mental, and Social Benefits of Practice-Based Movement

It's easy to think of movement as something that mainly shapes your body: your muscles, your joints, your endurance.

But for centuries, practices like yoga, dance, and martial arts have taught that movement is also a gateway to something deeper.

These traditions recognize that:

Your body and mind are not separate.

How you move shapes how you feel.

Shared practice creates connection, purpose, and belonging.

When you commit to engaged, lifelong practice, you discover that the benefits reach far beyond physical fitness.

Mind-Body Connection, Breath Coordination, and Nervous System Regulation

Many modern workouts focus on distraction—music blasting, screens glowing, timers beeping.

Practice-based movement is different. It draws your awareness back into your own body:

- The feeling of your feet pressing into the floor.
- The length of your breath as you move.

- The subtle shifts in balance and energy from moment to moment.

This mindful attention calms the nervous system.

Slow, deliberate breathing activates the parasympathetic response—reducing stress, lowering heart rate, and promoting recovery.

Over time, this carries into your daily life:

- You feel more centered in moments of frustration.
- You notice tension before it becomes pain.
- You learn to pause, breathe, and respond instead of react.

In a world that constantly pulls your attention outward, these practices bring you back to yourself.

Building Resilience, Confidence, and Mental Clarity

When you engage deeply with movement arts, you're not just training your body.

You're also cultivating:

Resilience

- Showing up, even when you don't feel motivated.
- Trying again after mistakes or setbacks.
- Trusting that progress comes from steady effort.

Confidence

- Learning new skills, no matter your age.
- Feeling competent and capable in your own skin.
- Proving to yourself that you can grow and adapt.

CHAPTER 10

Mental Clarity

- Letting go of distractions.
- Developing single-pointed focus.
- Experiencing moments of flow—where time disappears and only presence remains.

These qualities are not separate from fitness. They are the *foundation* that sustains it.

Community, Ritual, and Personal Meaning

One of the most overlooked benefits of these disciplines is the sense of belonging they create.

When you step onto a mat, into a studio, or onto a training floor, you join a lineage that stretches back generations.

You become part of a community that shares:

- Ritual: bowing in, warming up together, honoring teachers and each other.
- Language: the names of poses, steps, or techniques.
- Purpose: the quiet understanding that this is about more than exercise.

This shared commitment often becomes a source of deep meaning.

It reminds you:

You're not alone in your effort to grow.

At a time in life when many people feel isolated or disconnected, this connection is profoundly nourishing.

Why These Practices Nourish Beyond the Body

Ultimately, the greatest gift of movement arts is how they help you feel *more alive.*

More aware.

More compassionate toward yourself.

More engaged with the people around you.

They teach you that discipline can coexist with joy.

That structure can lead to freedom.

That mastery isn't measured in what you accomplish, but in who you become along the way.

Walk, Run, Swim, Bicycle

Sometimes the simplest forms of movement are the most powerful.

Walking, running, swimming, and cycling have been with us for millennia—not as "exercise," but as part of daily life and survival.

Today, they remain some of the most accessible ways to build strength, endurance, and mental clarity at any age.

These activities are also deeply aligned with **Applied Cognitive Fitness (ACF)** principles:

Use It to Improve It: You build capacity by doing.

Train with Purpose: Each session has a clear focus—distance, pace, technique.

Live with Stakes: Whether it's a brisk walk or a swim, you engage your body in ways that matter beyond the gym.

Perform Better Than You Practice: Over time, you notice how your training shows up in everyday life—carrying groceries, climbing stairs, staying steady on uneven ground.

Let's look at each of these timeless practices more closely.

Walking

History & Science:

Walking is our oldest form of locomotion. Some anthropologists believe it's the foundation of human endurance and brain development.

Modern research shows:

- Regular walking lowers all-cause mortality.
- It improves cardiovascular fitness, joint health, and mood.
- Even modest increases in daily steps (around 7,000–8,000) have significant benefits.

Psychology & ACF Connection:

Walking is also a moving meditation—a chance to unplug, reflect, and reconnect. It offers low cognitive load, making it an ideal space for mindful breathing and attention training.

How to Start:

- Aim for a daily walk, even if it's only 10 minutes.
- Vary the terrain if possible—grass, hills, sidewalks.
- Practice posture awareness and slow, steady breath.

Running

History & Science:

Running was once essential for hunting and migration. Today, it remains one of the most efficient ways to build aerobic capacity and resilience.

Studies show:

- Regular running improves VO_2 max and metabolic health.

- It supports bone density by applying controlled impact forces.
- Short, slow runs can be as beneficial over time as long distances.

Psychology & ACF Connection:

Running demands focus and presence. It's an opportunity to observe your self-talk and learn how to self-regulate under mild discomfort.

How to Start:

- If you're new, alternate walking and running in intervals.
- Focus on relaxed breathing and smooth, quiet steps.
- Use time rather than distance as your metric—start with 10–20 minutes.

Swimming

History & Science:

Cultures worldwide have practiced swimming for survival and sport for thousands of years. Unlike impact-heavy exercise, swimming is gentle on joints while providing full-body resistance.

Evidence shows:

- Swimming improves cardiovascular health and lung capacity.
- It builds muscle strength, particularly in the back and shoulders.
- Immersion in water can lower stress hormones and calm the nervous system.

Psychology & ACF Connection:
Swimming is uniquely immersive—literally and mentally. It demands rhythmic breathing, coordinated movement, and sensory focus, all core ACF principles.

How to Start:

- If you're not confident, consider adult swim lessons.
- Start with short sessions—5–10 minutes is enough to build comfort.
- Alternate strokes to engage different muscle groups.

Cycling

History & Science:

The bicycle revolutionized mobility and independence. Today, cycling is one of the most joint-friendly forms of cardio and strength training.

Research shows:

- Regular cycling improves leg strength, balance, and aerobic fitness.
- It supports mental health—outdoor cycling is linked to reduced depression and anxiety.
- It can be adapted to all fitness levels with adjustments in resistance and duration.

Psychology & ACF Connection:

Cycling blends steady aerobic effort with situational awareness, especially outdoors—navigating terrain, scanning for obstacles, and adjusting pace.

How to Start:

- Use a stationary bike if balance is a concern.
- Begin with 10–15 minute sessions at low resistance.
- Focus on smooth pedal strokes and upright posture.

Making These Practices Your Own

Whether you choose to walk, run, swim, cycle—or a combination—the most important thing is consistency.

These forms of movement don't require fancy gear or memberships. They meet you wherever you are:

- In your neighborhood
- At a community pool
- On a local trail or bike path
- In your living room, if you prefer a treadmill or stationary bike

A Closing Thought

It's easy to underestimate these simple activities because they don't look impressive on social media.

But over months and years, they build:

A resilient heart

A clear mind

A body that still loves to move

And they remind you that fitness doesn't have to be complicated to be life-changing.

Dance

If there is a single thread running through nearly every human society, it is the impulse to dance.

Before we had written language, before we built cities, we danced.

We danced to celebrate harvests, mark rites of passage, grieve losses, welcome seasons, tell stories, and simply feel alive.

Today, dance continues to be both ancient and modern—transcending borders, generations, and identities.

Whether you find yourself moving alone in your kitchen, learning folk steps at a cultural festival, or waltzing in a ballroom, dance is an expression of something essential:

The joy of inhabiting your body.

A Universal Human Practice

Anthropologists have documented dance traditions in every known culture, from the earliest archaeological records to the present day.

This universality suggests something profound:

Movement set to rhythm is not an optional part of being human.

It is how we connect—
with ourselves,
with each other,
with something greater than us.

Dance is where emotion, community, and vitality intersect.

Types of Dance

Dance takes many forms, and each offers unique benefits and experiences:

Social Dance
Ballroom, salsa, swing, tango—styles that emphasize partnership, connection, and improvisation.

Art Dance
Ballet, modern, contemporary—disciplines that train precision, grace, and expression.

Folk Dance
Circle dances, line dances, traditional steps passed down through generations—often performed in community celebrations.

Global Cultural Dance
Flamenco, hula, Bharatanatyam, African dance—each rooted in deep cultural heritage and storytelling.

There is no wrong place to start.
You can join a class, attend a festival, or simply put on music and move your body in your living room.

How Dance Fits in the ACF Model
Dance beautifully illustrates all seven ACF principles:

Use It to Improve It: Every session refines coordination, timing, and strength.

Learn What Matters: You focus on steps, rhythms, and patterns that challenge you in meaningful ways.

Train with Purpose: Each dance has its own goals—connection, expression, mastery.

Limit Passive Input: Dance requires active engagement; you can't phone it in.

Focus on Output: Your body becomes the instrument of the music.

Live with Stakes: The mild vulnerability of being seen and sharing movement adds energy and intention.

Perform Better Than You Practice: Skills learned in dance—balance, rhythm, adaptability—transfer to daily life.

Physical Benefits

- **Cardio Fitness:** Dancing at moderate intensity can significantly improve heart health and VO_2 max.
- **Strength:** Many styles train your core, legs, and stabilizers in dynamic ways.
- **Balance & Coordination:** Learning steps, turns, and transitions refines proprioception.
- **Flexibility:** Warm-ups and flows increase mobility.

Mental and Emotional Benefits

- **Cognitive Challenge:** Memorizing patterns strengthens memory and executive function.
- **Mood Elevation:** Dance reliably boosts endorphins and dopamine, reducing anxiety and depression.
- **Mindfulness:** When you are dancing, you are fully present—thinking less, feeling more.

Social and Cultural Benefits

- **Belonging:** Dance often happens in community, bridging generations and backgrounds.
- **Ritual:** It creates shared traditions and celebrations.
- **Identity:** Cultural dances connect you to heritage and collective memory.

How to Start

At Home: Put on your favorite music and move for 10–15 minutes without worrying about technique.

In Class: Look for beginner lessons in ballroom, Latin, line dance, or modern dance at local studios or community centers.

Online: Many instructors offer classes you can follow in your living room.

In Community: Attend cultural festivals, social dance nights, or folk dance groups—often welcoming and low-pressure.

A Gentle Reminder

You don't need to be "good" at dancing to benefit from it.

You only need to be willing to move.

The simple act of stepping into rhythm—alone or with others—is an ancient human birthright.

It is how generations have found courage, celebration, healing, and connection.

Yoga

If you asked ten people what yoga is, you'd probably get ten different answers:

A stretching routine

A philosophy

A spiritual practice

A form of exercise

A way to manage stress

And the truth is, they'd all be right—because yoga is vast.

It is one of humanity's oldest systems for integrating body, mind, and spirit.

CHAPTER 10

A Gentle Clarification

The kind of yoga most people encounter in gyms, studios, and community centers today is a branch called **Hatha Yoga.**

Hatha simply means "force" or "effort"—not in the sense of aggression, but of **consciously working with your body.**

It's the family of yoga that uses:

- **Physical postures (asanas)** to build strength, mobility, and balance
- **Breathwork (pranayama)** to calm and focus the mind
- **Relaxation** to restore and integrate

There are many sub-styles—some gentle and restorative, others athletic and demanding.

Gentle (Yin, Restorative, Kripalu)

Moderate (Hatha, Iyengar)

Dynamic (Vinyasa, Ashtanga, Power Yoga)

No matter which you explore, you can adapt it to your needs, abilities, and season of life.

Why Yoga is So Widely Practiced

Yoga's popularity is no accident. It offers something many modern fitness systems don't:

A built-in balance of effort and recovery

A holistic approach that includes nervous system health

A philosophy of self-study rather than self-judgment

Unlike competitive sports, yoga doesn't expect you to win.

It simply invites you to *come as you are,* and practice with sincerity.

How Yoga Fits with ACF Principles

Yoga is one of the purest expressions of the ACF model:

Use It to Improve It: Repeated practice gradually transforms mobility, stability, and awareness.

Learn What Matters: You study not just form, but *the quality of your attention.*

Train with Purpose: Each posture and breath is chosen intentionally.

Limit Passive Input: Distraction fades as you tune into sensation.

Focus on Output: Your body becomes the primary tool for learning.

Live with Stakes: Even simple postures can feel humbling, inviting humility and patience.

Perform Better Than You Practice: The calm and focus cultivated on the mat flow into daily life.

Benefits of Yoga for Lifelong Movement
Physical Benefits:

- Improved flexibility and joint health
- Better balance and fall prevention
- Increased muscle endurance and strength (especially in slower styles)
- Pain relief, particularly in the back and hips

Mental and Emotional Benefits:

- Reduced stress and anxiety
- Improved sleep quality
- Greater self-compassion and patience

Social and Community Benefits:

- Accessible classes almost everywhere
- Welcoming communities of all ages and backgrounds

How to Begin Without Overwhelm

If you've never tried yoga, start simple:

Try a gentle Hatha or Yin class. Many community centers and online platforms offer beginner sessions.

Focus on how it feels, not how it looks. Flexibility is not a prerequisite—it's a byproduct of practice.

Explore breath awareness. Even a few minutes of guided breathing can improve focus and reduce tension.

Be patient. Yoga rewards consistency, not intensity.

A Thoughtful Perspective

It's easy to think of yoga as "just stretching." But if you stay with it, you'll discover it's actually a way of relating to your body and mind.

A way of listening.

A way of respecting your own limits.

A way of discovering where effort meets ease.

And perhaps most importantly:

A way of remembering that you are not just a mind moving a body—you are a whole, living system worthy of care.

10.7 – Martial Arts

If you think of martial arts and picture only high kicks, flying throws, or sparring, you're not alone.

Martial arts can look intimidating from the outside—fast,

demanding, even confrontational.

But step inside any long-standing dojo or training hall, and you'll discover something very different:

People of all ages and abilities, practicing together.

A deep respect for elders and experience.

A culture where movement is lifelong, not limited to youth.

Like yoga, martial arts is a vast landscape.

It can be:

- A fitness practice
- A form of self-defense
- A competitive sport
- A cultural tradition
- A spiritual discipline
- Or any combination of these

There is no single "correct" reason to practice—only the commitment to show up with sincerity.

A Spectrum from Gentle to Dynamic

Many people are surprised to learn that martial arts includes some of the gentlest movement systems ever created:

Tai Chi and Qigong: Slow, flowing sequences designed to harmonize body and mind, improve balance, and cultivate internal energy.

Aikido: Circular, graceful techniques emphasizing redirection and non-resistance.

Karate, Taekwondo, Kung Fu: Striking arts ranging from athletic and powerful to precise and meditative.

Judo, Brazilian Jiu-Jitsu: Grappling disciplines with options for both competitive intensity and technical study.

Traditional Weapons Forms: Staff, sword, fan—practiced for coordination and cultural preservation.

No matter which path you choose, the heart of martial arts is the same:

Discipline, awareness, and the pursuit of personal growth.

How Martial Arts Fits with the ACF Model

More than any other movement tradition, martial arts naturally expresses the ACF principles:

Use It to Improve It: Skill only grows through repeated practice—there is no shortcut.

Learn What Matters: You focus on essential techniques, not flashy distractions.

Train with Purpose: Every drill, form, or sparring round has a clear intention.

Limit Passive Input: You can't check out mentally—your safety and progress depend on being fully engaged.

Focus on Output: Your body learns to apply power precisely, rather than randomly.

Live with Stakes: Whether you're practicing a self-defense technique or simply striving to master a form, there is always something at stake—your attention, your humility, your growth.

Perform Better Than You Practice: The discipline you build shows up everywhere—how you handle stress, how you carry yourself, how you meet life's challenges.

The Respect for Elder Practitioners

Perhaps more than any other movement tradition, martial arts celebrates the wisdom that comes with time.

It is not unusual to see:

- Masters in their 70s, 80s, or beyond demonstrating powerful techniques with quiet grace.
- Older students training alongside younger ones, embodying patience and depth.
- Dojos where seniority is not just about skill, but about character and dedication.

In many schools, it is expected that you will continue your practice until the end of your life.

This expectation isn't a burden—it is an honor.

It says:

Your worth is not in your speed or strength. It is in your willingness to keep showing up.

Benefits for Body and Mind
Physical Benefits:

- Improved balance and fall prevention (especially in Tai Chi and Aikido)
- Increased mobility and strength
- Enhanced coordination and reaction time
- Cardiovascular conditioning in more dynamic styles

Mental and Emotional Benefits:

- Greater focus and self-regulation
- Confidence in your ability to protect yourself if needed
- A sense of calm groundedness, even in stressful situations

Social and Cultural Benefits:

- Belonging to a lineage and community
- Shared rituals that foster respect and camaraderie
- Opportunities for intergenerational connection

How to Start Without Overwhelm

If you're new, consider:

Tai Chi or Qigong: Gentle, accessible, and often taught in community centers.

Beginner martial arts classes: Many schools offer low-pressure introductions focused on form and movement.

Watching a class first: Observing can help you understand the culture and see whether it feels like a good fit.

Asking questions: Most instructors will be glad to help you find an approach that suits your goals and abilities.

A Thoughtful Perspective

If you feel hesitant because martial arts seem too demanding or unfamiliar, remember:

You are not expected to fight or compete.

You are simply invited to explore.

To discover what it feels like to move with focus.

To study something bigger than yourself.

To join a tradition that honors discipline, respect, and lifelong learning.

Martial arts are not about conquering others.

They are about cultivating the steadiness and confidence to face life with an open heart—and a resilient body.

Movement Arts for a Lifetime

If you take only one message from this chapter, let it be this: **You don't have to stop moving as you age.**

You don't have to shrink your world, abandon curiosity, or surrender to the idea that vitality belongs to the young.

Yoga, dance, martial arts, swimming, walking, cycling—these are not just ways to stay fit.

They are invitations to keep learning, connecting, and expressing yourself in ways that nourish your body and spirit.

What Sets These Practices Apart

Unlike many sports or fitness trends, these lifelong movement arts:

Adapt to every season of life.

Your practice grows with you, becoming slower or deeper without losing meaning.

Value experience over performance.

You are not measured by how high you kick or how far you stretch, but by your sincerity and presence.

Offer community, ritual, and belonging.

They connect you to something larger than yourself—a lineage of people who have walked this path before you.

Train the whole self.

Every session blends body, mind, and emotion, creating benefits that ripple far beyond the hour you spend practicing.

A Respectful Invitation

Maybe you've always been curious about trying yoga.

Maybe you loved to dance when you were younger.

Maybe you've admired martial artists but assumed it was too late to start.

It isn't.

There is no "too late."
There is only this moment, and your willingness to explore.
You don't need to be strong, flexible, or experienced to begin.
You only need the openness to try.
Keep moving. Keep learning. Keep showing up.
Your body—and your spirit—will thank you.

Chapter 11

Integration, Adaptation, and Sustained Progress

Layering Your Lifestyle

By now, you've seen that sustainable fitness isn't about a single habit or heroic burst of motivation.

It's about **layers**—small choices stacked gently on top of each other until they create a life that supports your strength, mobility, and vitality without feeling forced.

If you've spent decades thinking of yourself as "not an active person," this can feel like a big leap. But here's the truth: no one is born with a perfect routine. No one wakes up one day with every habit in place.

This is a practice of gradual layering.

Turning Habits Into a Way of Life

In the beginning, movement might feel like something you *add* to your day—an appointment, a to-do. Over time, it becomes the backdrop. It becomes how you move through the world.

Maybe you start by walking after lunch. Then you notice you have more energy in the afternoon. That makes it easier to cook a nourishing dinner. Better food supports better sleep. And good rest makes you more likely to train the next morning.

One action feeds the next. That's layering in motion.

This isn't about perfection. You don't need to do everything every day. What matters is building a base layer that feels natural enough to sustain—especially when life gets busy or unpredictable.

Personalizing Your Fitness Strategy

No book—*not even this one*—can tell you exactly what your routine should look like.

Because you are the expert on your life.

Your season, your obligations, your health history, and your goals are unique.

So take what resonates here and make it your own.

Maybe your strategy includes:

- A brisk walk every morning before the day picks up speed
- Two resistance training sessions a week, even if they're short
- A Saturday dance class or swim that feels more like play than exercise
- A standing desk or mobility break every hour

Or maybe it looks different. That's not just acceptable—it's ideal.

Fitness at this stage of life is not a competition. It's a personal commitment to keep your body and mind engaged, supported, and nourished.

Progress Isn't Linear—And That's OK

One of the hardest lessons to accept is that progress does not move in a straight line.

Some weeks you'll feel energized, motivated, and capable of doing more. Other weeks, life will interrupt—illness, stress, family obligations, or just a body that needs extra rest.

This doesn't mean you're failing. It means you're human.

Fitness is a spiral, not a ladder.

You will revisit the same lessons. You will return to the basics. You will have seasons of growth and seasons of maintenance.

What matters is that you keep showing up.

When the momentum stalls, gently restart.

When doubt creeps in, remember why you began.

When you feel behind, remind yourself: **there is no behind**—only the next step forward.

A Gentle Invitation

If this feels like a lot, take a breath.

You don't have to have it all figured out today.

Just start with one layer—a daily walk, a weekly class, an extra glass of water. Practice showing up for yourself in small, consistent ways.

Over time, those small actions will grow into a lifestyle.

And that lifestyle is what will sustain your energy, your independence, and your confidence for the years ahead.

You're not building a fitness program.

You're building a life you can inhabit fully—one layer, one day, one decision at a time.

Chapter 11

Mindset for the Long Haul

If you remember nothing else from this book, remember this:

What you believe about aging shapes what is possible for you.

The research is clear: people who expect to decline often do so more rapidly. Those who expect to keep learning, moving, and engaging tend to preserve their strength, health, and independence far longer.

This isn't wishful thinking. It's biology.

Your beliefs influence:

How you perceive challenges

How motivated you feel to take action

How your brain and body respond to effort

If you start to see yourself as someone who *can* grow, adapt, and improve—at any age—you create the conditions to make it true.

Why Your Beliefs Matter So Much

Studies on aging have shown something remarkable:

People with a positive mindset about growing older live, on average, **7.5 years longer.**

Why?

Because beliefs drive behavior.

If you believe decline is inevitable, you're less likely to:

- Move your body regularly
- Try new things
- Challenge yourself
- Seek out supportive communities

If you believe you can continue to grow, you're more likely to:

- Invest in daily movement and strength
- Take care of your nutrition and rest
- Stay socially and mentally engaged

Over time, these small differences in action create big differences in outcomes.

Mental Rehearsal: Practicing Success Before It Happens

One of the most powerful tools you have is your imagination. Elite athletes, performers, and even surgeons use **mental rehearsal** to improve their skills and confidence.

You can use it too.

Before your next training session or walk, take a few moments to visualize:

- How it feels to move smoothly and confidently
- The sensations of strength, ease, and presence in your body
- The small victories—finishing a session, breathing steadily, feeling good afterward

Mental rehearsal helps your brain and nervous system prime themselves for success.

Over time, you stop seeing movement as a threat and start seeing it as something you are capable of and even enjoy.

Reflection: Learning from Every Experience

Another essential mindset practice is **reflection**.

Instead of judging yourself after a workout or a skipped session, ask:

- What worked well today?
- What felt challenging—and why?
- What would I like to try differently next time?

This gentle curiosity keeps you engaged without shame or guilt. Remember: you're not collecting data to criticize yourself. You're collecting data to keep learning.

Emotional Reinforcement: Feeling Good About Doing Good

Humans are wired to repeat behaviors that feel rewarding. That's why it helps to consciously **celebrate small wins**:

- Acknowledge when you complete a workout, even a short one.
- Notice when you feel a little stronger or more flexible.
- Take a moment to feel gratitude for your body and its capacity to adapt.

This isn't self-indulgent—it's practical. Positive emotion is the glue that helps habits stick.

The Psychology of Thriving at Any Age

At the heart of all of this is a simple question:
What story do you want to tell about your life?
One of decline and resignation?
Or one of curiosity, capability, and growth?
You don't have to pretend aging doesn't come with challenges. It does.

But you get to decide whether those challenges are the end of the story—or the beginning of a new chapter.

Linking to Cognitive and Emotional Health

Movement is often framed as something we do *for our bodies.*

But the truth is, it is just as vital for your mind.

Decades of research confirm what ancient traditions have always understood:

Physical training is one of the most powerful tools for sustaining mental clarity, emotional balance, and resilience as you age.

If you take nothing else from this chapter, remember this:

When you move your body, you are also training your brain—and your capacity to meet life with focus and steadiness.

How Training Supports Mental Clarity, Memory, and Focus

Every time you engage in purposeful movement, you're stimulating the parts of your brain responsible for:

Learning new information

Solving problems

Regulating attention

In fact, exercise has been shown to:

- Increase the size of the hippocampus (the brain's memory center)
- Improve executive function, helping you plan, organize, and adapt
- Boost neuroplasticity—the brain's ability to rewire and stay flexible

This is why so many people notice sharper thinking after a walk, a swim, or a dance class.

Movement literally fuels your brain with more oxygen, nutrients, and neurochemicals that help you feel clear and focused.

Emotional Regulation Through Movement and Physical Consistency

Exercise is often called nature's antidepressant—and for good reason:

It increases serotonin and dopamine, improving mood.

It reduces cortisol, the stress hormone that can cloud thinking and wear down your health.

It provides a healthy outlet for frustration, anxiety, or restlessness.

Even more importantly, **regular movement builds emotional resilience.**

When you practice showing up—especially when you don't feel like it—you teach yourself:

- That you can tolerate discomfort.
- That you can keep going even when motivation wavers.
- That you have tools to shift your state rather than be ruled by it.

Over time, these lessons accumulate into a quiet confidence that you can handle whatever life brings.

Lifespan Synergy: How Training Extends Capability Across Every System

The most exciting finding in modern science—and the most hopeful message of this book—is that movement creates **synergy across your lifespan.**

When you train your body, you also:

Improve metabolic health, reducing risk of diabetes and

cardiovascular disease

Protect bone density, reducing the chance of fractures

Enhance immune function, helping you recover faster

Support brain health, reducing the risk of dementia and cognitive decline

These benefits are not isolated.

They build on each other.

More strength leads to more independence.

More independence leads to more engagement.

More engagement leads to richer relationships, greater purpose, and deeper satisfaction.

This is why movement matters.

Not because it makes you look a certain way, but because it makes you **more able to live fully.**

In every decade of life, training is not just about staying fit. It is about **protecting the clarity and confidence you need to make the most of every day you're given.**

Conclusion

You're Not Done. You're Just Getting Started.

If you've read this far, it means something important:

You care about how you live.

You care about showing up for yourself—not just when it's convenient, but when it matters most.

You care about proving, to yourself more than anyone else, that **growing older doesn't mean growing smaller.**

Becoming the High-Functioning Version of Yourself

No matter where you started—whether you were active decades ago or have never had a regular practice—you now have the knowledge to begin building something new.

Not a perfect body.

Not a life free from challenge.

But a **high-functioning version of yourself**:

Strong enough to carry what matters—physically and emotionally.

Flexible enough to adapt when life changes course.

Confident enough to keep exploring, even when the path is

unfamiliar.

This is what real fitness means in your 50s, 60s, 70s, and beyond.

Not chasing youth, but honoring your capacity and expanding it, one choice at a time.

Aging as a Performance Advantage

One of the great secrets—rarely spoken in a world obsessed with novelty—is that age brings a kind of **quiet power.**

You already know how to be consistent.

You already know how to weather setbacks.

You already understand the value of patience and perspective.

These are the qualities that make training sustainable.

They are your performance advantage.

Youth may have energy and speed, but age has something deeper:

The wisdom of discipline.

You don't have to start over.

You only have to keep going.

A Gentle Invitation

So here, at the end of these pages, is your invitation:

Choose one place to begin.

One small action that feels possible today.

A walk after breakfast.

A gentle strength session.

A moment of stillness and breath.

Don't wait for the perfect moment.

Don't wait to feel completely ready.

Start where you are, with what you have, and trust that it will be enough.

A Closing Thought

You are not done.

You are not finished growing.

You are not out of time.

You are simply standing at the edge of a new chapter—one that only you can write.

You can fill it with movement, purpose, and the quiet pride of knowing you chose to keep becoming.

You're just getting started.

A Small Favor, If You Feel Moved

If this book has supported you, inspired you, or helped you see what's possible in your own life, I'd be deeply grateful if you'd consider leaving a review on Amazon.

Your thoughts—whether shared online or with a friend—help others discover these ideas and feel encouraged to begin their own journey.

Thank you for taking the time to read, reflect, and move forward. It means more than you know.

Appendix A

References and Resources

Below are selected books, articles, and online resources that informed the ideas in this book and can help you explore movement, nutrition, and cognitive vitality further.

General Fitness and Longevity

- **Peter Attia, MD** – *Outlive: The Science and Art of Longevity* A modern look at how exercise, nutrition, and medicine intersect to shape lifespan and healthspan. www.peterattiamd.com
- **Harvard Health Publishing** – *Exercise and Fitness After 50* A collection of evidence-based articles on cardiovascular health, strength training, and mobility for older adults. www.health.harvard.edu
- **American College of Sports Medicine** – *ACSM's Guidelines for Exercise Testing and Prescription* A professional reference (for those who want deep detail) on exercise standards.

www.acsm.org

Strength, Balance, and Mobility

- **National Institute on Aging** – *Exercise & Physical Activity: Your Everyday Guide*Simple guides to safe strength, balance, flexibility, and endurance training at any age.www.nia.nih.gov/health/exercise-physical-activity
- **Tai Chi for Health Institute** – Resources for learning Tai Chi as a lifelong balance and mobility practice.www.taichiforhealthinstitute.org

Cardiovascular Fitness

- **Zone 2 Training** – Learn more about aerobic base-building and why low-intensity cardio matters:www.foundmyfitness.com
- **VO_2 Max and Longevity** – *The Most Important Number in Aging* (Peter Attia Podcast)A layperson-friendly explanation of why aerobic capacity is a powerful predictor of lifespan.Listen here

Nutrition and Supplementation

- **National Institute on Aging** – *Healthy Eating*Balanced, non-dogmatic guidance on nutrition for older adults.www.nia.nih.gov/health/healthy-eating
- **Precision Nutrition** – A science-based platform with re-

sources on adapting nutrition to your goals and preferences. www.precisionnutrition.com
- **Examine.com** – In-depth analysis of supplements (creatine, vitamin D, omega-3s) with evidence grading. www.examine.com

Cognitive Fitness & Neuroplasticity

- **Applied Cognitive Fitness** by Jimmy LockettA foundational text for understanding how purposeful learning and engagement can improve brain function at any age.
- **Neuroplasticity After 60** – Key research findings on how the brain continues to adapt later in life.
- **The Synapse Project** – Landmark study on skill learning in older adults (Denise Park et al.)www.sciencedaily.com
- **National Institute on Aging – Cognitive Health**Evidence-based articles about lifelong brain health.www.nia.nih.gov/health/cognitive-health

Movement Arts and Lifelong Practice

- **Yoga Alliance** – Find a certified yoga teacher or program appropriate for older adults.www.yogaalliance.org
- **Dance for PD®** – An inspiring example of how dance supports vitality and resilience.www.danceforparkinsons.org
- **Martial Arts Resources**
- *Tai Chi: Moving for Better Balance* – CDC-supported evidence-based program.www.cdc.gov

- International Martial Arts Federation sites (varies by discipline)

Selected Scientific References

1. Salthouse, T.A. (2004). What and when of cognitive aging. *Current Directions in Psychological Science.*
2. Park, D.C., & Reuter-Lorenz, P. (2009). The Adaptive Brain: Aging and Neurocognitive Scaffolding. *Annual Review of Psychology.*
3. Erickson, K.I., et al. (2011). Exercise training increases size of hippocampus and improves memory. *PNAS.*
4. Borella, E., Carretti, B., & De Beni, R. (2008). Working memory training in older adults. *Applied Cognitive Psychology.*
5. Mather, M., & Carstensen, L.L. (2005). Aging and motivated cognition. *Trends in Cognitive Sciences.*

A Note on Personalization

This appendix is not a prescription—it's an invitation to explore. Before starting any new exercise, nutrition, or supplementation plan, please consult qualified professionals who understand your unique history and needs.

You don't have to use every resource here. Pick the ones that resonate, and remember: learning, movement, and growth are lifelong companions.

About the author

Jimmy Lockett has spent his life exploring the edges of human potential—through mental training, nutrition, music, movement, and stillness. A Juilliard-trained composer, and a 7th-degree black belt in Karate, Jimmy brings together two lifetimes of study into one integrated path.

As a performer and composer, Jimmy has appeared on Broadway, toured internationally, and had his works performed by orchestras and artists across the country.

For nearly six decades, Jimmy has studied and taught martial arts, including karate, jujutsu, judo, and Tai Chi, training under some of the most respected names in the world. He has also worked as a certified herbalist, paramedic, and shiatsu practitioner.

In the *You Can Still...* series, Jimmy blends modern neuroscience, ancient disciplines, and real-life experience into a dynamic roadmap for cognitive and physical vitality: the ability to grow mentally sharper, focus more deeply, learn more thoroughly, express more creatively, and continue to thrive at any age.